'This guide will be an invaluable resource for any young person receiving enhanced cognitive behavioural therapy (CBT-E) for eating disorders or considering this treatment. This guide intends to empower and equip a young person on their journey to recovery using a CBT-E approach. The book describes how eating problems develop and are maintained, and consequently how they can be successfully addressed. Taking part in CBT-E can be an effortful process, although the more effort a young person is able to put into therapy the more they are likely to benefit from it. This guide will help a young person to navigate this therapy and aid with challenges they might face along the way. It is also likely to be helpful for clinicians using CBT-E with young people, given its accessibility and deliberate efforts to translate any "jargon" into everyday terms.'

—**Rebecca Murphy, PhD,** *The Centre for Research on Eating Disorders at Oxford (CREDO), Department of Psychiatry, University of Oxford (UK)*

'Most eating disorder books are geared toward adults or parents—this is one of the first to be uniquely tailored for young people themselves. Brimming with relatable real-life examples, QR codes that link to helpful worksheets, and user-friendly descriptions of cutting-edge research, *A Young Person's Guide to Cognitive Behavioural Therapy for Eating Disorders* puts the patient in the driver's seat, encouraging them to play an active role in their own recovery. I can't wait to recommend this fantastic resource to all of my young patients receiving cognitive behavioural therapy for their eating disorder.'

—**Jennifer J. Thomas, PhD, FAED,** *Co-Director, Eating Disorders Clinical and Research Program, Massachusetts General Hospital, Associate Professor of Psychology, Department of Psychiatry, Harvard Medical School, President, Academy for Eating Disorders*

This book for young people receiving CBT-E for an eating disorder is an incredibly valuable and engaging resource. It comes alongside the young person and has the potential to "turbo charge" therapy by involving them as a fully informed and respected partner in the therapy.'

—**Tracey Wade,** *Matthew Flinders Distinguished Professor of Psychology, Flinders Institute for Mental Health and Wellbeing, Flinders University Services for Eating Disorder (Australia)*

'Clinical experience in the complex field of eating disorders has a priceless value, *A Young Person's Guide to Cognitive Behavioural Therapy for Eating*

Disorders makes available to young patients and their therapists a multi-year experience and all the knowledge of the authors about the use of this evidence-based therapy with the aim of empowering young people suffering from an eating disorder to fully benefit of this technique.'

—**Angela Favaro,** *Full Professor of Psychiatry—Department of Neuroscience, Padua University (Italy)*

A Young Person's Guide to Cognitive Behavioural Therapy for Eating Disorders

A Young Person's Guide to Cognitive Behavioural Therapy for Eating Disorders is a state-of-the-art guide for young patients struggling with disordered eating based on enhanced cognitive behavioural therapy (CBT-E).

CBT-E is one of the most effective treatments for eating disorders, including anorexia nervosa, bulimia nervosa and binge-eating disorder, which has recently been adapted for adolescents. Written by two experienced clinicians and clinical researchers working daily with teenagers suffering from eating disorders, and their parents, this book offers an effective mix of theory and clinical expertise that will appeal to all readers. The volume starts with a presentation the most current facts on eating disorders. Part 2 then provides young with eating disorders a complete description—accompanied by clinical examples and helpful vignettes on how to implement the main CBT-E procedures.

While this book is specifically tailored for young people aged between 15 and 25 years with eating disorders treated with CBT-E, it will also be useful for all young persons affected by eating disorders, and clinicians using CBT-E with young patients.

Riccardo Dalle Grave, MD is Director of the Department of Eating and Weight Disorders at Villa Garda Hospital, Verona (Italy). He has co-developed CBT-E for adolescents with eating disorders, recommended by many international guidelines.

Simona Calugi, PhD, is Clinical Research Director of the Department of Eating and Weight Disorders at Villa Garda Hospital. She has co-developed CBT-E for adolescents with eating disorders.

A Young Person's Guide to Cognitive Behavioural Therapy for Eating Disorders

Riccardo Dalle Grave and
Simona Calugi

Routledge
Taylor & Francis Group
LONDON AND NEW YORK

Designed cover image: © Getty Images

First published 2024
by Routledge
4 Park Square, Milton Park, Abingdon, Oxon OX14 4RN

and by Routledge
605 Third Avenue, New York, NY 10158

Routledge is an imprint of the Taylor & Francis Group, an informa business

British Library Cataloguing-in-Publication Data
A catalogue record for this book is available from the British Library

ISBN: 9781032378619 (hbk)
ISBN: 9781032378985 (pbk)
ISBN: 9781003342489 (ebk)

DOI: 10.4324/9781003342489

Typeset Times New Roman
by Apex CoVantage, LLC

Contents

About the authors

Riccardo Dalle Grave, MD, is Director of the Department of Eating and Weight Disorders at Villa Garda Hospital, Verona (Italy). His research within this department has addressed many aspects of eating disorders and obesity, including their diagnosis, assessment, maintenance mechanisms and treatment. In collaboration with Professor Christopher G. Fairburn, he developed an original inpatient treatment for eating disorders based entirely on enhanced cognitive behavioural therapy (CBT-E), and an adaptation of CBT-E for young people with an eating disorder. Dr Dalle Grave has a particular interest in assessing the effectiveness of CBT-E in adult and adolescent patients with eating disorders whose weight is very low, in both outpatient and inpatient settings. He is editor of the CBT-E website and Director of the Italian Advanced Training Course on the Treatment and Prevention of Eating Disorders and Obesity, which trains clinicians in cognitive behavioural therapy for eating disorders and obesity. He also supervises clinical CBT-E services across Europe, the USA, Australia and the Middle East. He is a fellow of the Academy of Eating Disorders and a member of the editorial boards of several scientific journals on eating disorders.

Simona Calugi, PhD, is Clinical Research Director at the Department of Eating and Weight Disorders at Villa Garda Hospital, Verona (Italy). Within this department, in collaboration with Dr Riccardo Dalle Grave, she is involved in assessing the efficacy of intensive enhanced cognitive behavioural therapy (CBT-E) and outpatient CBT-E for adults and adolescents. Dr Calugi's current research focuses on the effectiveness of CBT-E in treating adult and adolescent patients with eating disorders whose weight is very low, in both outpatient and inpatient settings, and studying specific and non-specific maintenance mechanisms of eating-disorder psychopathology. She is a member of the online CBT-E training group and on the teaching faculties of the Italian Advanced Training Course on the Treatment and Prevention of Eating Disorders and Obesity and several Italian cognitive behaviour-based psychotherapy schools. She is also President of the Italian Eating and Weight Disorder Association (AIDAP) and has extensive clinical experience delivering outpatient CBT-E to adult and adolescent patients with eating disorders.

Preface

This guide is not a self-help book. It is primarily intended for young people aged 15 to 24 undergoing enhanced cognitive behavioural therapy (CBT-E) for eating disorders. However, it would also be of interest to those undergoing other treatments or deciding which treatment would be best for them. If this applies to you, we suggest you skip ahead to the Letter to the Reader that follows this foreword.

The guide is designed to provide helpful information on eating disorders and describe the current strategies and procedures used in CBT-E to enable young people to overcome their illness. It will therefore also be useful for clinicians using CBT-E to treat young people or who are thinking of doing so. Anyone who wants to have up-to-date scientific information on eating disorders and innovative ways of treating them may also find it of interest.

CBT-E was initially developed at the Centre for Research on Eating Disorders at Oxford (CREDO) for adults with eating disorders. It is a flexible and personalised psychological treatment based on the "psychological model" explanation of eating disorders. It originates from the observation that the main features and maintenance mechanisms of the different diagnostic categories of eating disorders (e.g., anorexia nervosa, bulimia nervosa, binge-eating disorder and similar states) are essentially the same. Hence, if these maintenance mechanisms can be interrupted in a specific eating disorder, it should be possible to interrupt them by similar means in other eating disorders. This strategy, which has been borne out by the research into CBT-E, is known as a "transdiagnostic approach" to eating disorder treatment.

Thanks to the success of CBT-E in clinics around the world, the idea of adapting to make it suitable for young people was raised about 15 years ago at the Villa Garda Hospital Department of Eating and Weight Disorders in Italy, based on our experience that young patients with eating disorders display the same specific eating-disorder features as adults. This observation suggested that young people could also benefit from addressing the psychological and behavioural features and maintenance mechanisms of eating disorders via CBT-E, especially following the adaptations introduced to suit adolescents and young adults.

In fact, it is usually in in mid-adolescence that eating disorders take root, and people of this age have the highest hospitalisation rates for eating disorders. Without rapid and effective intervention, the symptoms may persist for ten years or more, with many young people requiring intensive and effective community treatment until they reach their mid-twenties and beyond. Despite this, child and adolescent mental health services have traditionally been separated from adult mental health services, which attempt to treat eating disorders using different strategies and procedures. This division creates a discontinuity in the care process at a crucial time in a young person's treatment and can precipitate deterioration of their illness. Furthermore, only a few patients treated for eating disorders by child and adolescent eating disorder services receive treatment from adult eating disorder services after the age of 18, which increases the risk of relapse and may even result in premature mortality.

As CBT-E is designed to treat all eating disorders across the age spectrum, it offers the concrete possibility of implementing a treatment that overcomes some of the difficulties encountered in more fragmented conventional services. Moreover, the research indicates that about two-thirds of young patients who complete CBT-E achieve lasting remission of their eating disorder. Such promising findings have influenced international health policy, and the 2017 National Institute for Health and Care and Clinical Excellence (NICE) guidelines for eating disorders (evidence-based recommendations for health and social care services and professionals) recommend cognitive behavioural therapy (CBT) for young people with any form of eating disorder.

Although manuals have been published to guide clinicians and parents through the implementation of CBT-E, this is the first set of guidelines to be published specifically aimed at young people (aged 15 to 24) undergoing the treatment. It explains clearly what eating disorders are, what CBT-E entails, and how to make best use of CBT-E strategies and procedures. The Extra Information section at the back contains a brief description of the broad form of CBT-E, which is used to treat people with more complex forms of eating disorders, and how CBT-E can be optimally adapted for remote (online) delivery. As a major goal of CBT-E is for the patient to be cognisant of and actively involved in their own treatment, this guide can be considered essential reading.

Acknowledgements

We would like to take this opportunity to thank our esteemed colleague Christopher Fairburn, whose ideas inspired us to write this book. Particular thanks are also due to Anna Forster for editing the English text and helping to make our technical information comprehensible to non-experts. Last, but by no means least, we would like to extend our heartfelt gratitude to the patients we have had the privilege to support; they not only inspire our work but have also made invaluable suggestions that have enabled us to become better therapists and to perfect the guidance presented in this book.

Letter to the reader

Dear Reader,

Transitioning from childhood to adulthood is full of daunting challenges, even in the best of circumstances, but when you suffer from an eating disorder, it can be terrifying and even more confusing. Indeed, eating disorders have a profound impact on your physical, psychological and social wellbeing. Their effects can be devastating and long-lasting, so it is essential to treat them early and effectively.

If you are suffering from an eating disorder, you may be feeling helpless, hopeless and lost. Take heart, however, in the knowledge that by picking up this guide, you may have already set yourself on the right path to healing. It is designed to help you understand what we know about eating disorders, but above all to guide you through a treatment that has been scientifically proven to be effective in the majority of cases. We are talking about enhanced cognitive behavioural therapy (CBT-E for short), which the experts agree is as effective as or more effective than any other treatment available for eating disorders. For this reason, the major international guidelines recommend CBT-E for people with eating disorders.

It is therefore likely that you have already been referred for CBT-E, and that this book has been recommended to you by your therapist. However, it is also possible that you have not yet decided which treatment to undergo and are weighing up your options, or that another treatment you have tried has failed to produce the results you wanted. Whatever the case, this guide is filled with the information you need to understand your eating disorder and practical suggestions on things you can do to aid your full recovery. We have done our best to use language that is easy for most young people to understand, but it is important that you and your therapist have a shared language so that you can communicate effectively. For this reason, there are some technical terms included in **bold**—these are explained in simple language in the Jargon Buster boxes. If you are confused about some of the concepts or procedures explained, do not hesitate to ask your therapist.

Indeed, not having the right information can result in people with eating disorders having misconceptions about the causes of their problem and may prevent you from dealing with it quickly and efficiently. Armed with misleading information, you may waste precious time undertaking therapy that is not right for you and is therefore unlikely to help you recover. It may even make things worse. For this reason, Part 1 of this guide gives you a detailed overview of the most up-to-date scientific knowledge on eating disorders. You should read this section carefully and take time to process the information before choosing a treatment or starting CBT-E. Part 2 of the book sets out the various stages of a CBT-E programme, what each will involve and what you can do to make the most of this opportunity to return to a healthy, happy life.

In fact, your engagement and involvement will be crucial to the success of CBT-E, so it is important that you have a clear understanding of what is happening to you and how the treatment seeks to help you get better. You might be tempted to dive straight into Part 2, but this would be a mistake—Part 1 (Chapters 1 to 5) contains information essential for working effectively with your CBT-E therapist and putting you on the right road to recovery.

For example, did you know that people with different eating disorders (anorexia nervosa, bulimia nervosa, binge-eating disorder, etc.) all have similar patterns of thinking and behaving? CBT-E exploits this by helping you to learn to think and behave more healthily. This is what cognitive behavioural therapy means. CBT-E targets the processes that "cement" the way a person with an eating disorder thinks, and consequently behaves, making it easier to break the vicious cycles that lead to and prolong their illness. It is a tried and tested approach that has been improved thanks to many years of dedicated scientific research (which is why we call it "enhanced"). It differs from other forms of treatment offered to young people with an eating disorder (some of which you may already be familiar with) because its underlying aim is to empower you to change rather than to force change upon you. You will be in charge of your progress at all times, and your therapist will never ask you to do anything that you do not agree to do. Their job will be to help you understand and show you, step by step, how to overcome the destructive or unhealthy behaviours that are likely making your life a misery.

Every person is unique, and CBT-E has been designed to be flexible. This means it is suitable for everybody, no matter their age, individual diagnosis or the severity or duration of their illness. This is backed up by the science. Many rigorous clinical trials have proven that CBT-E is one of the most effective forms of treatment for all types of eating disorders in young people. About two-thirds of young patients who complete the treatment get well and stay well. If you strive to consistently apply the strategies and procedures that you learn, and make the treatment a priority, there is no reason why you should not be one of them.

This guide is essentially a roadmap of CBT-E. Its purpose is to give you the facts you need to successfully navigate the three steps of treatment and the modules it contains. Your therapist will the act as your "tour guide," but you will be in the driving seat. Young people who have used this book to support their CBT-E journey in the past have said that knowing what the treatment will entail before they started helped them engage and feel in control. They found Part 1 of this guide especially useful, as a reliable source of information about eating disorders and the treatment itself. They also stated that it was helpful to have the book on hand as a practical guide and reminder on how to apply treatment procedures between sessions.

We hope that you too will find it helpful, and that it provides all the knowledge you need to recover from your eating disorder.

Best of luck on your journey!

Riccardo and Simona

Part 1

Understanding eating disorders

1

What is an eating disorder?

Anorexia nervosa and bulimia nervosa are terms that you probably know but may not really understand. The media tends to paint a simplistic picture of eating disorders, and most people think that the terms "anorexic" and "bulimic" mean being underweight and eating large amounts of food, respectively. However, they are in fact much more complex disorders that have profound effects on both mind and body. This chapter explains the real meaning of these terms and discusses why it is better to consider eating disorders as a single disorder, rather than many distinct disorders.

Eating problem or eating disorder?

Most people diet or **binge** in their lives, but this does not mean that they are "anorexic" or "bulimic." In other words, they do not have an eating disorder. Their diet is not extreme or overly strict, or their binges are occasional and do not have lasting consequences on their physical health and quality of life. This is therefore nothing to worry about. Persistent over- or undereating may become "problematic" but likely does not require specialist treatment, as it is just a phase and will return to normal on its own. Indeed, an "eating problem" is not the same as an "eating disorder." By definition, a disorder is an illness or condition that has a negative impact on normal physical or mental functioning. Thus, people whose diet is so extreme or rigid, or whose bingeing is so frequent, that it worsens their health, wellbeing or quality of life are classed as having an eating disorder.

> JARGON BUSTER
>
> **binge** (verb): to do something, especially eating or drinking, to excess

According to the current way of thinking in the medical community, there are three main eating disorders:

1. Anorexia nervosa
2. Bulimia nervosa
3. Binge-eating disorder

DOI: 10.4324/9781003342489-2

However, the research shows that many people, especially young people, with an eating disorder do not fall neatly into one of these three categories. There are several terms used to describe these people's eating disorders, but for the purposes of simplicity, in this book, we will refer to them as "other eating disorders."

Anorexia nervosa

Anorexia nervosa was the first eating disorder to be described, in 1694 by the English physician Richard Morton. At the time, it was considered a rare disease, but it is now known to be much more common. Anorexia nervosa mainly afflicts young women, but about one in eight cases occurs in males. In fact, the research indicates that about 1.4% of females and 0.2% of males will suffer from anorexia nervosa during their lives. It is more commonly seen in white populations, but the number of cases appears to be growing worldwide, particularly in Asia and the Middle East.

For an individual to be said to have anorexia nervosa, two main conditions must be met:

1. The person should be **significantly** underweight, and this should be due to their efforts, rather than any other cause.
2. The person should show evidence of placing excessive importance on their shape, weight or both—they become one of or the most important things in their lives. Their self-esteem depends mainly, or even totally, on their ability to control their shape and/or weight. Therapists call this the "overvaluation" of shape and weight, and this is described in detail in Chapter 3.

> JARGON BUSTER
>
> **significantly** (verb): to a large, notable or important degree

Rather than being worried about their low weight, people with anorexia nervosa are terrified of gaining weight and becoming fat. For this reason, they are often said to have a "morbid fear of fatness" or a "weight phobia," and their dieting and other weight-control behaviours are driven by a "relentless pursuit of thinness."

When girls and women lose too much weight, this often causes their periods to stop (the medical term for this is "amenorrhea"). However, this no longer needs to occur for a diagnosis of anorexia nervosa to be made, as some underweight people may show all the psychological features of anorexia nervosa but still have regular periods. Besides, it does not apply to girls whose period have not yet started, those taking the contraceptive pill or, of course, males. However, the loss of periods in a girl should always be considered a possible warning sign of anorexia nervosa (after pregnancy is ruled out).

People with anorexia nervosa reach a low weight by eating very little and sometimes exercising excessively. They tend to avoid the foods they consider fattening, and in some cases, they may even fast. About a third also "binge" frequently, but at these times do not often eat what would normally be considered an excessive amount of food (which is why we call these episodes "subjective binges"). Binge-eating episodes differ from overeating or "stuffing your face" in that the person suffering them loses all control over their eating—they may want to stop but feel unable to. In such cases, the binges are often followed by one or more "compensatory behaviours" to make up, or compensate, for the lapse and to help them lose the weight that they (wrongly) think they have put on during the binge. These compensatory behaviours used to "undo" the damage done by the binge may include excessive exercising and/or fasting or even more restrictive dieting, but often take the form of **purging**, i.e., making themselves sick (which we call "self-induced vomiting") or taking laxatives and/or diuretics (water pills).

JARGON BUSTER

purge (verb): to use laxatives, diuretics or self-induced vomiting in the (futile) attempt to rid the body of unwanted food

Fast Fact

Purging is pointless as well as potentially dangerous, as it does not actually make you lose weight. See Chapter 4 for the science.

Some young people with anorexia nervosa get better after a short period of therapy or without any treatment. However, if they don't, they may require prolonged and complex specialised treatment. Without effective treatment, a lifelong condition known as "severe and enduring" anorexia nervosa may develop, which occurs in about 10–20% of people. In these cases, the disorder continues to harm a person's health and quality of life to a greater or lesser degree.

Interestingly, *about half of people who initially present with anorexia nervosa develop bulimia nervosa* (a phenomenon called "migration") or another eating disorder—put a pin in this information for later ( ).

Bulimia nervosa

The term bulimia nervosa was introduced in 1979 by Professor Gerald Russell of the Maudsley Hospital of London in his scientific paper *Bulimia nervosa:*

An ominous variant of anorexia nervosa. A lot of research from 1980 onwards has shown that this disorder mainly affects young women. However, bulimia nervosa can develop in people of any age, gender, race or background. The proportion of males with this disorder is uncertain, but it is probably less than one in ten cases. The research indicates that about 1.9% of females and 0.6% of males suffer from bulimia nervosa during their lifetime.

To qualify an individual for a diagnosis of bulimia nervosa, the person must not meet the criteria for anorexia nervosa (see above) *at that time* (📌) and must display the following three features:

1. Experiencing recurrent objective (not subjective) binge-eating episodes. These episodes involve the person eating what is normally considered a large amount of food in a short period of time and are accompanied by a sense of loss of control over eating (a feeling that they cannot stop eating or control what or how much they are eating). These episodes are typically secretive and followed by intense feelings of guilt and shame.
2. After the objective binge-eating episodes, engaging in one or more extreme compensatory weight-control behaviours, including purging, overdosing on slimming pills, excessive exercising, extreme dieting or fasting.
3. Overvaluing the importance of shape, weight or both (see earlier).

On average, binge-eating episodes and inappropriate compensatory behaviours are required to occur at least once a week for three months to receive a diagnosis of bulimia nervosa.

Bulimia nervosa usually begins in the late teenage years with the adoption of extreme and strict dietary rules motivated by excessive concerns about shape and weight (overvaluation). In about a quarter of cases, there has been a period in which the person qualifies for a diagnosis of anorexia nervosa (see the criteria above). However, after a certain time, the diet is periodically interrupted by binges followed by compensatory behaviours such as self-induced vomiting, laxative **misuse**, strict dieting and/or excessive exercising. This vicious cycle of dietary restriction, bingeing and compensatory behaviours rarely produces a lasting calorie deficit. This explains why people with bulimia nervosa are typically in the normal weight or overweight range.

> JARGON BUSTER
>
> **misuse** (verb/noun): use (something) in the wrong way or for the wrong purpose

Once established, the so-called diet–binge–purge cycle makes bulimia nervosa hard to shift: it becomes self-perpetuating, although the severity may vary. Without effective treatment, bulimia nervosa may persist. More than 20% of people with the disorder suffer the effects on their health and quality of life for long periods of time. However, *about 20% of individuals with bulimia nervosa are later diagnosed with binge-eating disorder or another eating disorder* (📌), while migration to anorexia nervosa is less frequent.

Binge-eating disorder

The main feature of binge-eating disorder is, of course, binge-eating episodes. Although people with obesity experiencing recurrent binge-eating episodes were described by Professor Albert Stunkard of the University of Pennsylvania as far back as 1959, the official diagnosis is a recent one. Indeed, it was not until the mid- to late 1980s, when research into the **prevalence** of bulimia nervosa in the community found that many people who met the diagnostic criteria for the disorder did not regularly practice compensatory behaviours after binge-eating (no self-induced vomiting, misuse of laxatives or fasting, etc.). Hence, a new diagnostic category had to be defined.

> JARGON BUSTER
>
> **prevalence** (noun): the commonness, or amount of people in a population with a certain condition or disease at a specific time

To qualify an individual for a diagnosis of binge-eating disorder, two features must be present:

1. Recurrent objective binge-eating episodes (as described for bulimia nervosa)
2. No regular use of compensatory behaviours

The second excludes bulimia nervosa, which involves compensatory behaviours. To qualify for a diagnosis of binge-eating disorder, binge-eating should occur, on average, at least once a week for three months.

It typically starts in late **adolescence** or early adulthood, and it is the most common eating disorder in young people. However, it can develop at any age, and about 2.8% of women and 1.0% of men have this disorder in their lifetimes. Unlike anorexia nervosa and bulimia nervosa, in which the female to male ratio is 9:1, binge-eating disorder is spread more evenly, with approximately four males getting it for every six females. The disorder has a similar prevalence across all ethnic/racial groups. In general, people affected are younger, and most are not overweight.

> JARGON BUSTER
>
> **adolescence** (noun): the phase of life between childhood and adulthood (10–19 years of age)

Unlike anorexia nervosa and bulimia nervosa, which usually start with strict dieting, binge-eating disorder often begins with objective binge-eating episodes. These are frequently linked to stressful events. As binge-eating often results in weight gain; this leads some people to make several attempts to lose weight. In most cases, however, their diet is so irregular (binge–diet–binge), that they cannot achieve lasting weight loss.

> JARGON BUSTER
>
> **onset** (noun): the start or time when a disease manifests

In some cases, the **onset** of binge-eating disorder does occur after a period of strict dieting. However, people with binge-eating disorder tend to eat a lot with little control, which distinguishes them from those with bulimia nervosa, who are able to stick to an excessive and restrictive diet between binges.

People with binge-eating disorder tend to be very distressed about their binge eating, which is usually accompanied by shame and self-criticism. They generally experience a long history of binge-eating episodes, which often increase in frequency during periods of stress. They also, however, experience long periods without bingeing, and it often goes away on its own (spontaneous **remission**). In those who do not achieve remission, migration to anorexia nervosa or bulimia nervosa is rare, but obesity and depression are common.

> JARGON BUSTER
>
> **remission** (noun): the symptoms get better or disappear

Other eating disorders

As mentioned, there are other eating disorders of clinical severity, i.e., that require treatment, but do not meet the diagnostic criteria for anorexia nervosa, bulimia nervosa or binge-eating disorder. These eating disorders have been given various names (including eating disorders not-otherwise-specified, unspecified eating disorders, atypical eating disorders and, more recently, other specified or unspecified feeding or eating disorders). Here we use the broad term "other eating disorders."

The "other" presentations are much more common than previously thought. Indeed, they have been found in about one-fifth of people with eating disorders who seek treatment. In other words, *20% of eating disorder patients do not fit into the three main diagnostic categories* ( ). As with anorexia nervosa and bulimia nervosa, other eating disorders are most common in young women. However, males and adults may also suffer from these disorders. The available data indicate that about 1.5% of people will develop one of these disorders during their lifetime.

The category of other eating disorders can be divided into five more or less distinct subgroups:

- **Atypical anorexia nervosa:** meets all the criteria for anorexia nervosa, except that, despite significant weight loss, the individual's weight is within or above the normal range.
- **Bulimia nervosa (of low frequency and/or limited duration):** meets all the criteria for bulimia nervosa, except that binge eating and inappropriate compensatory behaviours occur, on average, less than once a week and/or for less than three months.
- **Binge-eating disorder (of low frequency and/or limited duration):** meets all the criteria for binge-eating disorder, except that the binge eating occurs, on average, less than once a week and/or for less than three months.
- **Purging disorder:** recurrent purging behaviour to influence weight or shape (e.g., self-induced vomiting, misuse of laxatives, diuretics or other medications) but no objective binge-eating and not underweight.
- **Night-eating syndrome:** recurrent episodes of night eating, i.e., eating excessively after the evening meal or in the middle of the night. People who get out of bed to eat need to be aware of and remember doing so (not sleepwalking) to be diagnosed with night-eating syndrome. The night eating causes significant distress and/or makes daily functioning difficult.

Not much research into these other eating disorders has been done, so little is known about their **course**, but it is thought that about 60% of those affected will recover. In most cases, they begin in adolescence or early adulthood, and about *one-quarter to one-third of individuals have a history of anorexia nervosa and/or bulimia nervosa* (📌).

> JARGON BUSTER
>
> **course** (noun): the behaviour of an illness over time

Eating disorders in young people

Young people with eating disorders have essentially the same psychological features as adults (see Chapter 3). However, young people are more likely to exercise excessively and less likely to binge eat than older adults. Some adolescents do not seem to overvalue their shape and weight, but instead place too much importance on their control over eating. Eating disorders are particularly worrying in teens, as they become so focused on their eating (or weight or shape) that they do not form healthy relationships with their peers. Not only does this have a negative impact on their quality of life, it also affects their cognitive development and prevents them "growing up" properly and becoming fully independent from their parents.

The physical consequences of eating disorders also tend to be more severe in younger people. Teens are particularly vulnerable to the effects of under-eating and weight loss because their organs are not yet fully developed. In particular, there are three physical complications that require special attention (see Chapter 4):

1. Brittle bones
2. Stunted or delayed growth
3. Structural and functional changes in the brain

There is still not much definitive data available on the distribution of eating disorders in adolescence. However, anorexia nervosa is the most common disorder, followed by the other eating disorders, while bulimia nervosa and binge-eating disorder are seen less often. During the 2019 coronavirus pandemic (COVID-19), the number of new cases of eating disorders dramatically increased, most among female teenagers. To give you an idea of the size of the problem, the infographic shown in Figure 1.1 reports the age distribution of the patients seeking treatment for outpatient CBT-E in our clinic at Verona before and during the COVID-19 pandemic.

As far as treatment is concerned, there is some good news: younger people generally recover more quickly from their eating disorder than adults do.

Eating disorders in males

Although eating disorders are much more commonly seen in females, they have been observed in males since 1689, when Dr Richard Morton described the first documented case of anorexia nervosa in a young man. Nowadays, it is usually reported that, on average, 10% of people with anorexia nervosa are male, although this may be an underestimate. Indeed, boys and men are less likely to be aware of having an eating disorder and are often more reluctant to seek help.

Another problem is that the questionnaires and interviews used to assess for eating disorders have been specifically designed for women, and we may not be asking the right questions for detecting eating disorders in boys and men. For example, a question like "I frequently check my muscles," is not usually asked during an eating-disorder exam, while others like "I think my thighs are too large" are. This reflects one of the main differences between males and females with eating disorders, namely body image concerns. While the primary concern of women and girls with an eating disorder is being too fat, males tend to be concerned about not having enough muscle mass. This is probably why males with eating disorders are more likely to use excessive exercise than purging for weight control, even after binges. In addition, while

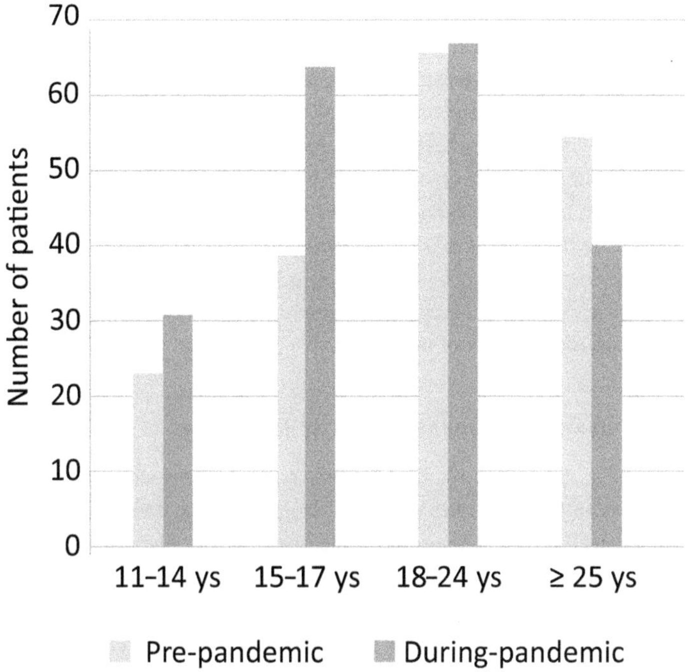

Figure 1.1 The age distribution of patients seeking treatment for outpatient CBT-E before (01/01/2018 – 08/03/2020) and during (09/03/2020 – 31/12/2021) the COVID-19 pandemic

Source: Reproduced with permission from Dalle Grave, R., Calugi, S., Sartirana, M., Chignola, E., Franchini, C., Macrì, L., . . . Morandini, N. (2022). Number and characteristics of patients seeking treatment for eating disorders at a CBT-E clinical service before and during the COVID-19 pandemic. *IJEDO*, 4, 30–33. doi:10.32044/ijedo.2022.06. This work is licensed under a CC BY 4.0 license.

females with eating disorders often avoid high-calorie food items, males tend to tailor their diet to muscle-building, increasing their intake of proteins and creatine supplements, perhaps even resorting to misuse of steroids, growth hormones and other substances. Obviously, these are sweeping generalisations, but it appears that what is recognised as the "relentless pursuit of thinness" in females manifests in males as the "relentless pursuit of muscularity." However, some males report, as the females, a morbid fear of weight gain and a marked desire for thinness.

Although there is little data available (due to the lower number of cases reported), a history of obesity (about 50%), depression, substance misuse (drug and alcohol abuse) and/or suicidality is more common in males with anorexia nervosa than in the general male population. Roughly 20% of males with an eating disorder identify as homosexual, but this may be due to under-reporting by heterosexual males. Indeed, even if they are aware that they need help, males are less likely to seek treatment for their eating disorder, likely due to gender stereotypes and the idea that eating disorders are something that only affect women. When males do finally go to the doctor about their eating disorder, they have often been ill for a long time, which makes it more difficult for them to recover.

However, males with eating disorders manifest the same medical complications as females, and CBT-E is flexible enough to be tailored to the individual. Hence, it also works well in males, as features of eating disorders such as excessive exercise and checking of muscle mass can be tackled effectively, irrespective of the gender of the patient.

Eating disorders in gender minority population

Once again, the data is scarce, but early reports have indicated that there are significantly higher rates of both eating disorders and attempted suicide among LGBTQ+ people than among their heterosexual and cisgender peers. This finding has recently and dramatically been confirmed by the Trevor Project, which surveyed 34,759 young LGBTQ+ people, recruited between October and December 2020 via targeted ads on social media. The Trevor Project found that 9% of LGBTQ+ people aged 13 to 24 reported that they had been diagnosed with an eating disorder. This rate is much higher than that previously found in studies of lifetime prevalence in both adolescents aged 13–18 (3%) and young adults aged 18–29 (5%) in the general US. population. Eating disorders were even more prevalent among transgender boys/men and non-binary young persons assigned female at the birth (AFAB). What is more, young LGBTQ+ people who had ever been diagnosed with an eating disorder had nearly four times greater odds of attempting suicide in the past year than those who had never suspected nor had an eating disorder diagnosis. It has been proposed that the higher rates of eating disorders and suicide risk among LGBTQ+ people are mainly related to their reported experiences of bullying and discrimination, as well as internalised stigma and having to hide their LGBTQ+ identity. However, CBT-E can be adapted to the specific need specific of the gender minority population. In particular, the treatment can address in a personalised way the sociocultural pressure to have a lean body shape and the interpersonal difficulties related to coming out, experiencing harassment and discrimination that often contribute to the maintenance of the eating disorder psychopathology and obstacle the change among the LGBTQ+ people.

The reality: is there only one eating disorder?

If you have been making a note of the pins we dropped earlier, you may already be having doubts about the medical classification of eating disorders into several distinct diagnosable illnesses. Indeed, there are at least three major problems with this distinction:

JARGON BUSTER

biomarker (noun): a measurable indicator of some biological state or condition

1. There are no specific **biomarkers** for eating disorders. In other words, there is nothing we can measure to determine whether you have an eating disorder, or which eating disorder you may have.
2. Eating disorders share most clinical features.
3. Eating disorders frequently migrate from one to another.

As we shall see next, these observations indicate that it is extremely unlikely that the medical classification of eating disorders is an accurate description of the clinical reality.

Eating disorders lack specific biomarkers

The medical classification bases the distinction between eating disorders on behavioural (e.g., binge eating, purging, excessive exercising, etc.) and psychological features (e.g., overvaluation of shape and weight), not on biological alterations. In other words, we cannot test your blood sugar levels or DNA for eating disorders as we can for other medical diseases. In short, there is no biological evidence to support the current distinction between eating disorders.

Eating disorders share most clinical features

Most people with eating disorders report similar eating habits and concerns about shape and weight (see Chapter 3). For example, overvaluation of some kind or another is seen across the board and is accompanied by behaviours like extreme dieting, fasting, bingeing, purging and/or excessive exercising to various degrees and in varying combinations. This means that the distinction between the various eating disorders is often difficult to make and, in any case, appears artificial. For example, if we follow the medical classification, a young person with the characteristics of bulimia nervosa and a body mass index (BMI) of 18.49 (the minimum threshold is 18.5), will receive a diagnosis that will depend on her weight, rather than the clinical characteristics of the disorder. If her weight is considered significantly low, she will receive a diagnosis of anorexia nervosa, otherwise bulimia nervosa. Another common problematic comparison is between bulimia nervosa and binge-eating disorder diagnoses. In people who do not vomit or do not misuse laxatives, the distinction between the two disorders is determined by the amount of food that the person eats between binge-eating episodes. If the amount is small, they will receive the diagnosis of bulimia nervosa, otherwise binge-eating disorder. In other words, the boundaries between the various diagnostic categories of eating disorders are often unclear.

Fast Fact

BMI, or body mass index, is calculated by dividing body weight by height squared, and is expressed in units of kg/m^2. For example, a person who weighs 50 kg (110 lb, or just under 8 stone) and is 1.65 m tall (5'4") has a BMI of 18.38 kg/m^2. Anything below 18.5 kg/m^2 is considered underweight in people aged 15 or over.

Eating disorders migrate from one diagnosis to another

Several studies assessing the course of eating disorders have found that they often migrate between different diagnostic categories, but only rarely to other mental illnesses. It is not uncommon to see people given one specific eating disorder diagnosis (e.g., anorexia nervosa) and then another (e.g., bulimia nervosa), even over the course of a year. This diagnostic migration usually happens without a significant change in the major, or core, psychological features, namely the overvaluation of shape, weight, eating and/or their control.

It is our conviction that it is not the disorder that is changing, but that instead it the presentation of a single eating disorder that has transformed. This is backed up by our clinical experience, in which we have encountered numerous people who in adolescence had received a diagnosis of anorexia nervosa that then migrated to bulimia nervosa, or sometimes another eating disorder later on. This is illustrated by the example case that follows: one of our patients who received diagnoses of three different eating disorders throughout her life.

Example case
Three eating-disorder diagnoses or one single eating disorder?

Jenny (not her real name) received a diagnosis of anorexia nervosa at the age of 14. By that point she had lost a significant amount of weight, from 54 kg to 38 kg. She told her family doctor that she was terrified of gaining weight, and that she was constantly preoccupied with her shape and weight, which were the most important things in her life (overvaluation). Her periods had also stopped, and her doctor correctly diagnosed that she was presenting anorexia nervosa.

However, at the age of 15, she broke one of her own dietary rules and started binge eating and self-inducing vomiting afterwards. Her body weight increased to 55 kg and her periods returned to normal. Nonetheless, she was still showing signs of overvaluation of shape and weight and was therefore diagnosed with bulimia nervosa.

At the age of 17, she stopped self-inducing vomiting after bingeing, and her weight rose to 65 kg. As she continued to binge and display overvaluation of shape and weight, however, her diagnosis was changed to binge-eating disorder.

According to the medical classification, the patient had three specific eating disorders at three separate times. Do you think that this is, in fact, the case, or did she have a single disorder with characteristics that changed over time?

The transdiagnostic perspective

Bearing in mind the above, Prof. Fairburn and his colleagues at Oxford University (UK) were unconvinced by the official medical classification. They thought that it would be better to consider eating disorders as a single diagnostic category with different presentations, rather than a class of several distinct conditions (see Figure 1.2). This is called the "transdiagnostic perspective," or view, of eating disorders.

Adopting a transdiagnostic perspective has important implications for the treatment of eating disorders. If we think, as the official medical classification suggests, that there are several different eating disorders, it follows that there should be a specific treatment for each. If, however, the Oxford University team is correct, and there is a single eating disorder that persists and may evolve (but likely not into another psychological disorder), there must be a treatment capable of treating patients with all its major presentations. This is, in fact, the case, as CBT-E has been shown by the research to be equally as effective in anorexia nervosa, bulimia nervosa and binge-eating disorder. This is because it targets the processes that act to reinforce or cement the psychology of people with all categories of eating disorder. These processes are what we call "maintenance mechanisms," which drive the conscious and subconscious decisions of people with eating disorders and are the same whether the person is diagnosable with anorexia nervosa, bulimia nervosa or binge-eating disorder, whether typical or atypical. More on these maintenance mechanisms

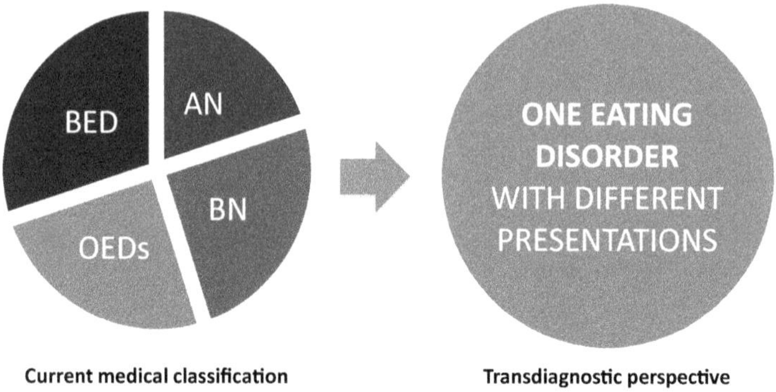

Figure 1.2 Schematic representation of how eating disorders are classified by the current medical classification, and by the transdiagnostic perspective

Note: AN = anorexia nervosa; BN = bulimia nervosa; BED = binge-eating disorder; OEDs = other eating disorders

in Chapter 3, but for now be aware that CBT-E, which specifically targets them (as described in Chapter 5), works in both adolescents and adults, no matter their eating disorder diagnosis.

In Summary

- People who adopt an extreme and rigid diet and/or binge so frequently that it *impairs their physical health and/or quality of life* are said to have an eating disorder.
- The official medical classification distinguishes between three main eating disorders, namely anorexia nervosa, bulimia nervosa and binge-eating disorder.
- Many people with an eating disorder do not fall into these three categories and have therefore been grouped into the category "other eating disorders."
- There are no specific biomarkers for eating disorders.
- The clinical features of eating disorders are largely, whether the person is adult or adolescent, regardless of their gender identity or sexual orientation. However:
- The physical complications of eating disorders tend to be more severe in adolescents than adults, and teens are also more likely to exercise excessively, but less likely to binge eat.

- Males with eating disorders are also more likely to exercise excessively, the goal being to become muscular rather than thin (as is more usual in females).
- Eating disorders frequently migrate from one diagnosis to another.

• Take-home message

The scientific evidence supports the transdiagnostic perspective of eating disorders, i.e., that they should be considered as different presentations of a single disorder, and CBT-E, being "made-to-measure," works equally well in each.

Further reading

American Psychiatric Association. (2013). *Diagnostic and statistical manual of mental disorders, (DSM-5)*. Arlington, VA: American Psychiatric Publishing.

Dalle Grave, R., & el Khazen, C. (2022). *Cognitive behaviour therapy for eating disorders in young people: A parents' guide*. London: Routledge.

Fairburn, C. G., Cooper, Z., & Shafran, R. (2003). Cognitive behaviour therapy for eating disorders: A "transdiagnostic" theory and treatment. *Behaviour Research and Therapy*, *41*(5), 509–528. doi:10.1016/s0005-7967(02)00088-8

Galmiche, M., Dechelotte, P., Lambert, G., & Tavolacci, M. P. (2019). Prevalence of eating disorders over the 2000–2018 period: A systematic literature review. *American Journal of Clinical Nutrition*, *109*(5), 1402–1413. doi:10.1093/ajcn/nqy342

Murray, S. B., Nagata, J. M., Griffiths, S., Calzo, J. P., Brown, T. A., Mitchison, D., . . . Mond, J. M. (2017). The enigma of male eating disorders: A critical review and synthesis. *Clinical Psychology Review*, *57*, 1–11. doi:10.1016/j.cpr.2017.08.001

Nagata, J. M., Ganson, K. T., & Austin, S. B. (2020). Emerging trends in eating disorders among sexual and gender minorities. *Current Opinion in Psychiatry*, *33*(6), 562–567.

Treasure, J., Duarte, T. A., & Schmidt, U. (2020). Eating disorders. *Lancet*, *395*(10227), 899–911. doi:10.1016/s0140-6736(20)30059-3

2

Why did I get an eating disorder?

The short answer to this is *we don't know*. There are lots of ideas and theories regarding the causes of eating disorders floating around the media and social networks. However, they are often wildly incorrect and lack a solid scientific basis. Recurrent questions asked by our young patients are: "Are eating disorders caused by a bad relationship with my parents or my mom?"; "Is it due to social pressure to be thin?"; "Is it a personal choice or a disease?"; "Is it a call for help or a protest?" There are no simple answers to these questions. The reality is that we are only just beginning to home in on the causes of eating disorders. However, we now have a better understanding of somc factors that seem to increase the risk of developing eating disorders. Ultimately, these may help us to design effective prevention strategies for these disorders, but for now they can only help guide treatment.

Potential risk factors for eating disorders

> JARGON BUSTER
>
> **incidence** (noun): occurrence, rate or frequency

The increase in the **incidence** of anorexia nervosa after the 1960s, the appearance of bulimia nervosa in the 1980s and the dramatic rise in the incidence of eating disorders among young people during the COVID-19 pandemic (see later in this chapter) suggest that social factors play an important role. However, the fact that only some individuals develop eating disorders, despite being subjected to the same social conditions as those who don't, indicates that some other individual processes are involved.

The variety of potential causes of eating disorders makes researching them very complicated. As saw in the previous chapter, these disorders are not always easy to identify, which makes the situation even more difficult (see Chapter 1). Even the same eating disorder will develop and evolve differently in different people and often coexist with other mental disorders, like

DOI: 10.4324/9781003342489-3

anxiety or depression. All these factors make it very difficult to design robust research into the causes of eating disorders and the effectiveness of treatments. However, the data we have today indicates that they seem to arise from a combination of genetic and environmental risk factors. Future research will be necessary to discover how these genetic and environmental factors interact, and thus how eating disorders arise and develop.

Genetics

The **heritability** of eating disorders has been calculated indirectly through studying families or twins. Current research uses sophisticated and complex genetic testing methods to identify which genes may be responsible. What we have found so far is that female relatives of people diagnosed with anorexia nervosa are 11 times more likely to develop it than relatives of individuals without anorexia nervosa. Twin studies—looking at the incidence of eating disorders among genetically identical people—have estimated that anorexia nervosa heritability ranges from 28% to 74%. However, this broad variability is a reflection of the problems with definitive diagnosis of anorexia nervosa mentioned earlier. If different criteria are being used to diagnose a disorder, it is impossible to come up with an accurate, specific figure.

> JARGON BUSTER
>
> **heritability** (noun): the extent to which genetics influences a trait or disorder

This is where genetic research comes in. In the search for the biological alterations that have not yet been identified, the DNA of 16,692 people with anorexia nervosa from 17 countries was tested and compared with the DNA of 5,525 controls without anorexia nervosa. Nowadays, the technology allows us to rapidly scan complete sets of DNA belonging to many people to find genetic variations that may be linked to a particular **trait** (like blue eyes, for example) or disease. The hope is that by comparing the genes of people with and without an eating disorder, we will discover which genes, or sets of genes, may be involved.

> JARGON BUSTER
>
> **trait** (noun): distinguishing quality or characteristic

Thus far, eight **genetic variants** associated with anorexia nervosa have been identified. There appear to be significant genetic links with other mental disorders, like obsessive-compulsive disorder, depression, anxiety and schizophrenia, but also with physical activity,

> JARGON BUSTER
>
> **genetic variant** (noun): permanent change in DNA sequence (aka "mutation")

metabolism and body measurement traits. If you remember your biology lessons, metabolism is the process by which the body converts food into energy. This indicates that anorexia nervosa could be a mental *and* metabolic disease. However, we still need to determine the meaning of these genetic variations and how they interact with other factors to cause anorexia nervosa.

As for the other eating disorders, a similar study is being done on people with binge spectrum disorders. These seem to have slightly lower levels of heritability than those found in anorexia nervosa (35–45%), and genetic links with alcohol problems and obesity.

Psychological processes

Psychology researchers have come up with specific theories to explain how eating disorders arise and evolve. Among these, cognitive behavioural theory is the one that has influenced treatment the most. The theory holds that dieting—the behaviour seen at the start of most eating disorder onsets—can lead to eating disorders in certain individuals (likely those with a genetic predisposition) through two main mechanisms. This is not to say that dieting in itself causes the eating disorder, but it is the door through which an eating disorder can enter. When we ask our patients about the start of their eating disorder, we always find that they fit into one or both of the following two categories:

1. A person who has a general need to feel in control of various aspects of their lives, like school, work or sports performance. When they shift their efforts towards controlling their eating, they may be at risk of their diet becoming overly strict. These are people whose attempts to control the uncontrollable may "open the door" to an eating disorder. They run the risk of becoming a "control freak" about eating control, as they place too much importance on it, something we call *overvaluation of eating control*.
2. A person who places great importance on their body shape and weight, as they have internalised something called the "social thin ideal." This is the idea that a woman should be slender and shapely, and a man should be lean and muscular. These are people who are chasing an impossible dream and may leave the door open to an eating disorder in the process. Because they have internalised the thin ideal, they place too much importance on their shape and weight, something known as *overvaluation of eating control*.

This is how an eating disorder develops (see the flow chart in Figure 2.1). Subsequently, other processes begin to operate and contribute to the persistence of the eating disorder, which we will discuss in detail in Chapter 5.

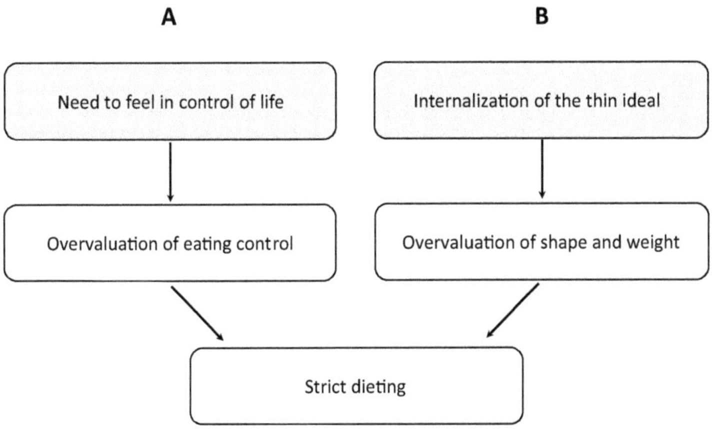

Figure 2.1 The two ways eating disorders develop, according to cognitive behavioural theory

Source: Reproduced with permission from *Cognitive Behaviour Therapy for Eating Disorders in Young People: A Parents' Guide* by Riccardo Dalle Grave & Carine el Khazen, Copyright © 2021 Taylor and Francis.

Other risk factors

Researchers have identified several other factors that may put people at risk of developing an eating disorder. These potential risk factors differ in nature and specificity. Some are risk factors for psychological problems in general, like childhood trauma such as sexual abuse or complications with birth. Other factors put you at risk of eating disorders specifically. These include early experiences of fat-shaming and weight-bullying, which can trigger dieting and negative feelings about food and eating, such as sadness, fear and loneliness. This makes it more likely that an eating disorder will develop. Some factors have been identified as specifically increasing the risk of bulimia nervosa. These include childhood and parental obesity, early puberty and having alcoholic parents. Others are more specific to anorexia nervosa, such as a low weight before the dieting that triggers the eating disorder is begun.

Finally, some personality traits put you more at risk of developing an eating disorder. The first of these is low self-esteem, which is common in all eating disorders. The second is perfectionism, which is frequently seen in individuals who will go on to develop anorexia nervosa (see Table 2.1).

Table 2.1 Some potential risk factors of eating disorder identified by research

General risk factors

- Being female
- Being an adolescent or young adult
- Living in a Western society or in a country influenced by Western culture

Individual risk factors

Having family members with the following conditions:

- Eating disorders
- Clinical depression
- Alcoholism
- Obsessive and perfectionistic traits
- Obesity

Experiencing the following before the development of the eating disorder:

Adverse parenting (especially low contact, high expectations, parental discord)

- Family dieting
- Obstetric/perinatal complications
- Sexual abuse
- Fat-shaming and weight-bullying
- Professional or recreational activities that encourage thinness (e.g., sports or modelling)
- Dieting
- Obesity
- Low weight (even prior to weight loss)
- Eating and digestive problems in early childhood
- Concerns about body weight and shape
- Certain personality traits (low self-esteem, perfectionism, mood intolerance)
- Negative internal experiences, such as sadness, fear and/or loneliness

In summary

The causes of eating disorders are still not well known. Available data indicates that they seem to arise from a combination of genetic and environmental risk factors, but how these factors interact is unclear. This means that we do not know how to prevent eating disorders.

The cognitive behavioural theory holds that dieting that characterises the onset of many eating disorders in certain individuals has two main origins:

- The first is a need of control of life, which gets displaced onto controlling eating.
- The second is the presence of overvaluation of shape and weight in individuals who have internalized the "thin ideal."

• Take-home message

Talking to patients indicates that the mechanism triggering an eating disorder is strict dieting caused by overvaluation of shape and weight and/or overvaluation of eating control. These processes are therefore valid targets for treatment.

Further reading

Fairburn, C. G., Cooper, Z., & Shafran, R. (2003). Cognitive behaviour therapy for eating disorders: A "transdiagnostic" theory and treatment. *Behaviour Research and Therapy*, *41*(5), 509–528. doi:10.1016/s0005-7967(02)00088-8

Lie, S. Ø., Rø, Ø., & Bang, L. (2019). Is bullying and teasing associated with eating disorders? A systematic review and meta-analysis. *International Journal of Eating Disorders*, *52*(5), 497–514. doi:10.1002/eat.23035

Mitchell, J. E., & Peterson, C. B. (2020). Anorexia Nervosa. *New England Journal of Medicine*, *382*(14), 1343–1351. doi:10.1056/NEJMcp1803175

Schaumberg, K., Zerwas, S., Goodman, E., Yilmaz, Z., Bulik, C. M., & Micali, N. (2019). Anxiety disorder symptoms at age 10 predict eating disorder symptoms and diagnoses in adolescence. *Journal of Child Psychology and Psychiatry*, *60*(6), 686–696. doi:10.1111/jcpp.12984

Treasure, J., Duarte, T. A., & Schmidt, U. (2020). Eating disorders. *The Lancet*, *395*(10227), 899–911. doi:10.1016/s0140-6736(20)30059-3

Watson, H. J., Yilmaz, Z., Thornton, L. M., Hübel, C., Coleman, J. R. I., Gaspar, H. A., . . . Bulik, C. M. (2019). Genome-wide association study identifies eight risk loci and implicates metabo-psychiatric origins for anorexia nervosa. *Nature Genetics*, *51*, 1207–1214. doi:10.1038/s41588-019-0439-2

3

Psychological and behavioural features of eating disorders

Eating disorders can change a young person's normal, happy life into a miserable one. They make people think and behave in ways that are both debilitating and self-perpetuating, trapping the individual in a downwards spiral that damages their physical and mental health and may stretch their relationships with parents, siblings and friends to the breaking point. As mentioned in the previous chapter, eating disorders (as conceptualised by the official medical classification) share psychological and behavioural features, which can be displayed in various combinations. This chapter details the typical ways that people with eating disorders think and behave, describing the vicious cycles that these psychological and behavioural features create and the ways in which they disrupt people's lives.

The main psychological and behavioural features common to eating disorders are the following:

- Overvaluation of shape, weight and eating
- Preoccupation with shape, weight and eating
- Fear of gaining weight or getting fat
- Feeling fat
- Extreme dieting
- Binge-eating episodes
- Excessive exercising
- Self-induced vomiting
- Misuse of laxatives and/or diuretics (aka water pills)
- Body checking/avoidance

Events, moods, emotions and other psychological issues can affect how people with eating disorders think and behave, and these are discussed at the end of the chapter.

Overvaluation of shape, weight and eating control

I am obsessed with my weight and how thin my legs and belly are. I'm never satisfied with my appearance. Nothing else matters to me and I feel low and worthless

DOI: 10.4324/9781003342489-4

because I don't like what I see in the mirror. I must get thinner—if I put on so much as a pound (half a kilo) I get desperate.

While most people judge themselves based on their relationships with other people and how they perform at school or in sports, for example, people with eating disorders base their self-evaluation mainly, or even entirely, on their body weight and shape, and their ability to control these. This form of self-evaluation, called *overvaluation of shape and weight*, is considered the primary, or core, psychological feature of eating disorders. This is because it is common to most people with eating disorders but is rare in the general population. In addition, it is the driving force behind most other eating disorder features, whether directly or indirectly.

It is essential here to distinguish between the overvaluation of shape and weight and *body dissatisfaction*—a term we commonly use to describe a dislike of our own physical appearance. Body dissatisfaction is common in the general population but, in most cases, is not a medical problem, as people who are unhappy with their appearance generally have other things in their lives that make them feel happy or proud of themselves. Because their self-esteem is based on several things—what we mental health professionals call *life domains*—it does not overly affect their quality of life. This stands in stark contrast to people with an eating disorder, whose "prime directive," to be thinner or weigh less, has a damaging effect on their physical and psychological wellbeing.

The easiest way to think about life domains is to imagine a pie chart. Usually, people have several interests that give them self-satisfaction and make themselves feel good about themselves. These people will have several roughly equal slices in their pie—the bigger the slice, the more importance the person gives to that life domain. As you can see from Figure 3.1, the pie chart

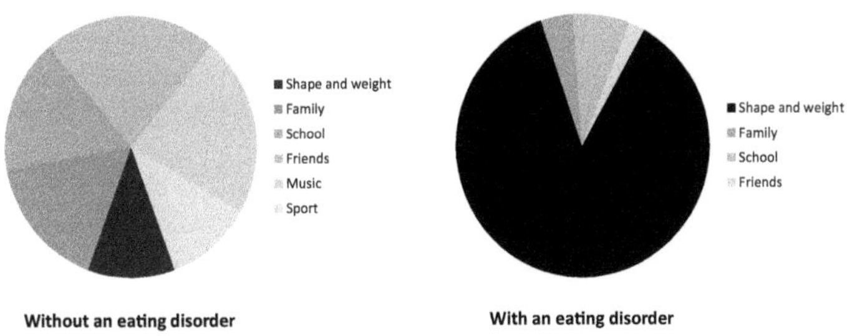

Figure 3.1 Graphical representation of the self-evaluation scheme of teens without and with an eating disorder

Source: Reproduced with permission from *Cognitive Behavioural Therapy for Adolescents with Eating Disorders* by Riccardo Dalle Grave & Simona Calugi Copyright © 2020 The Guilford Press.

of a person with an eating disorder looks very different. They are so preoccupied with their shape and weight that their pie has one massive slice and only thin slivers representing the other life domains (schoolwork, family, friends, sports, etc.). This is a good illustration of how much an eating disorder can affect someone's life.

Fast Fact

Sometimes people with eating disorders are less concerned with their shape and weight and more concerned with the need to exert control over eating. In other words, it is not so much the result as the process that drives them. We say that the core psychological feature of eating disorders in these people is the *overvaluation of eating control*. This means that their self-worth is mainly based on their ability to control what, how, when and where they eat. This feature often **coexists** with the *overvaluation of shape and weight*, but not always.

> JARGON BUSTER
> **coexist** (verb): exist in the same place or at the same time

Why is overvaluation unhealthy?

There are four main reasons why overvaluation makes it difficult to achieve a healthy, balanced self-evaluation and is damaging to the health and wellbeing of an individual:

1. *Basing self-esteem on one life domain is risky*. Indeed, when a person with an eating disorder fails to control their shape, weight or eating, their entire self-evaluation system collapses. In other words, it is like having all your eggs in one basket.
2. *It never leads to success*. With overvaluation, it is impossible to be skinny enough or attain the "perfect" body shape or eating control. In other words, the basket that is being used to hold the eggs is full of holes.
3. *It marginalises other important life domains*. If your basket is full of eggs, there is no room for anything else. In the same way, overvaluation leaves little room for the other important areas of life (e.g., school, relationships, hobbies) that generally contribute to a balanced, stable and healthy self-evaluation system.
4. *It leads to unhealthy behaviours*. As we shall see later in this chapter, the things that people with overvaluation do in the attempt to achieve their

"prime directive" are physically and psychologically damaging. Their efforts create a downward spiral of misery and ill health.

The easiest way to see the effect that overvaluation has on life is to imagine that, instead of slices of a pizza, life domains are represented by legs on a stool; a stool with one enormous leg and a few little legs will not hold you up for long, if it can even stand upright at all! A self-evaluation system with balanced legs—one that allows for various types of interests, successes and rewards—will be much more comfortable and far less fragile.

Preoccupation with shape, weight and eating

I'm always worrying about my looks and constantly compare myself with people who are thinner than me. I think about eating all day, every day: when I'm at school, when I'm out with my friends, and even when I'm watching a movie. I can't get my weight out of my mind.

A direct consequence of judging yourself only or mainly on your shape, weight or eating is that you can think of little else: this we call *preoccupation with shape, weight and eating*. A little stress may help you solve problems when they are short-lived, and your concerns are focused on overcoming appropriate, real and objective challenges. For example, being worried about your grades may prompt you to study that much harder for a school exam, and therefore get a better result. However, if the problem you are concerned about cannot actually be solved, there is no way out or relief. As people who strive to overcome the biological urge to eat and change their natural body weight will never achieve their goals, they will never be free of their concerns. When this occurs, we say that the person has become stuck in an *eating-disorder mindset.*

What is the effect of the eating disorder mindset?

1. People with an eating-disorder mindset have a peculiar way of looking at themselves and others.
2. For example, they may only notice thin people, or those with a flat stomach or big muscles. They don't even see that there are plenty of other people around who are as "imperfect" as them, or that the slimmest, prettiest girl at their gym is thoroughly unpleasant, for example. By only focusing on people who are "better" than them in some way they think of as important, they cannot have an unbiased view of the world, which will inevitably make them very unhappy.
3. Negative emotions associated with an eating-disorder mindset include anxiety and apprehension about the ability to control eating or lose weight, an intense fear of gaining weight, and feelings of guilt and mood swings related to perceived failures. These may even intensify efforts to diet and

other extreme weight-control behaviours, leading to a vicious circle that it is impossible to escape from.

4. The eating-disorder mindset often leads to other specific behaviours, such as constant body checking or body avoidance (see later in this chapter). But dwelling on a specific part of the body (such as a "flabby" tummy) or avoiding situations where it is normal not to be covered up from head to foot (e.g., going swimming or to the beach) themselves amplify preoccupation with shape, weight and eating control. Sometimes, the signals get so scrambled that a person mislabels negative sensations or emotional experiences as "feeling fat." In other words, normal feelings no longer have normal meanings—being angry, sad, tired, gassy or frightened is the same as feeling fat. As the eating-disorder mindset leaves little room for positive emotions or experiences, the end result is that the person "feels fat" 24/7, even if they are, in fact, severely underweight.

Fear of gaining weight or getting fat

> *I am absolutely terrified of gaining weight. I can't even look at certain foods for fear of getting fat! I skip meals and weigh myself three times to try to reassure myself that I'm not putting on weight, but it seldom makes me feel any better.*

Another direct consequence of the overvaluation of shape and weight is the *fear of gaining weight or becoming fat*. This fear does not lessen, even if you lose, or have already lost, a significant amount of weight. In fact, the fear of gaining weight tends to increase as the weight drops off and the eating-disorder mindset becomes locked in place.

Why is anorexia nervosa not a phobic disorder?

The fear of getting fat or putting on weight is not the same thing as a weight phobia. Think of someone with claustrophobia: that is the irrational fear of confined spaces. If they are put in a tight space, they will feel a very narrow range of emotions from severe anxiety to outright terror. They usually know on some level that their fear is excessive, but they can do nothing about it, so as a result they avoid lifts (elevators) or other small spaces so as not to feel those negative emotions. However, they generally do not report feeling euphoria or a sense of power when they are not in confined spaces.

In contrast, people with anorexia nervosa, although they may feel unreasonably afraid of getting fat, tend to report that their efforts to control weight give them a sense of triumph, mastery, self-control and superiority. Especially in the early phases of their weight loss, patients often say they feel "happy," "exultant," "satisfied," "powerful" and "proud" as they see their weight going down. They often see weight loss as a goal, achievement, virtue and/or a source of pleasure.

With this mindset, they see concerns about shape, weight and eating, and even the associated anxiety or stress, as useful tools to help them keep control over their shape and weight. Rather than weight phobia, then, it is the overvaluation of shape, weight and eating that is driving and reinforcing the eating disorder. Like most of its other clinical features, fear of putting on weight stems from this specific core psychological feature.

> WANT MORE SCIENCE? SEE:
>
> Dalle Grave, R., Sartirana, M., & Calugi, S. (2019). Weight phobia or overvaluation of shape and weight? A cognitive analysis of the core psychopathology of anorexia nervosa. *IJEDO*, *1*, 57–60. doi:10.32044/ijedo.2019.08

Feeling fat

> *I feel fat every time I weigh myself or look in the mirror. I also feel fat when I am tired, sweaty or sad. If I feel fat, it means that I am fat. It makes me want to try even harder to lose weight.*

Feeling fat is an experience reported by many young people, but the intensity and frequency of this feeling appear to be far greater among those with eating disorders, whether they are underweight, normal weight or overweight. There has not been very much research on feeling fat in eating disorders. Remarkably little has been written about it, although the term is used in many languages worldwide.

Feeling fat is not an emotion like being happy, sad, afraid, surprised or angry, or a physical sensation like feeling full or bloated. It is not linked to the actual state of the body, as it fluctuates in intensity from day to day, and even throughout the day. Obviously, body weight does not change so much within such a short timeframe. Therefore, feeling fat appears to be the result of mislabelling other experiences. These may include body awareness (e.g., receiving comments on appearance, body checking, physical contact, being sweaty, body wobbling, tight clothing), adverse physical states (e.g., feeling bloated, premenstrual, full, hungover, sleepy) and **aversive** emotional states (e.g., feeling depressed, lonely, bored, unloved). To put it simply, they confuse feeling bad or strange with feeling fat.

> JARGON BUSTER
>
> **aversive** (adjective): causing a strong dislike or avoidance

How does feeling fat maintain eating disorders?

Feeling fat tends to be equated with being fat by people with an eating disorder, whether they are overweight or not. It therefore seems to be the expression of excessive concerns about shape and weight. Feeling fat maintains the eating disorder by reinforcing shape dissatisfaction and prompting dieting. It feeds into the overvaluation of shape and weight by increasing preoccupation with shape and weight, and therefore also eating.

Extreme dieting

> *After I'd been dieting for about three months, I couldn't stop thinking about food. I was so terrified that I would put the weight back on again that my diet got even stricter.*

Most people with an eating disorder, unless it is binge-eating disorder, follow an extreme diet. Rather than adopting general heathy-eating guidelines, they set themselves multiple, demanding and precise dietary rules to limit what they eat. This "extreme dieting" has three main characteristics:

1. It is excessively strict, in that it involves the adoption of several dietary rules requiring continuous vigilance and constant commitment.
2. It is inflexible, in that the rules adopted must always be followed to the letter.
3. It is persistent, and the dieting does not stop even when one becomes underweight.

Such a rigid attitude to dieting is driven by the overvaluation of shape and weight, or by a need to maintain strict control over eating. This is different from the normal desire to lose those extra pounds or to prevent weight gain.

It is essential at this point to distinguish between two aspects of extreme dieting, *dietary restraint* and *dietary restriction*, as both are unhelpful and therefore need to be addressed during CBT-E.

Dietary restraint

Dietary restraint is a term used to describe the attempt to restrict what you eat. While many people without eating disorders adopt moderate and flexible dietary restraint to control their body weight and eating, those with an eating disorder self-impose dietary rules that are extreme and rigid. By "extreme" we mean numerous, overly strict, demanding and inflexible. Typically, a person exhibiting extreme dietary restraint will have many self-imposed rules to follow, involving when (e.g., never before/after 6 pm), how much (e.g., less than X number of calories a day) and what to eat (e.g., only fruits and vegetables). They feel the need to stick rigidly to all of these rules at all times in order to maintain a feeling of being in control.

The dietary rules of people with eating disorders are often associated with various forms of *food checking*, such as repeatedly reading labels on the calorie composition of foods, weighing food several times, counting the calories to eat and checking what others eat (especially those who eat little). As we shall see, it is also the type of dieting that encourages binge-eating episodes.

Dietary restriction

Dietary restriction is a term used to define true undereating in the biological sense. Some people with eating disorders say they do this because they are not hungry, but this is rarely true. Indeed, except in people with major depression, loss of appetite is seldom the leading cause of food limitation, which instead is seen a goal to be actively pursued.

As they are not providing their body with enough fuel, the person inevitably loses weight, often a significant amount, but also develops specific physical and psychosocial symptoms caused by undernutrition. The next section, "Low Weight and Starvation Symptoms," describes these in some detail, but, generally speaking, people who are focused on extreme dieting tend to find that they lose control in other areas of life. Their work performance or grades may slip because they find it difficult to concentrate, and their interpersonal relationships may suffer because it makes it difficult to eat with others. They become anxious before and during eating due to the fear of not being able to follow their extreme dietary rules, and crushing guilt and shame when this inevitably occurs.

How does extreme dieting maintain the eating disorder?

As we mentioned at the beginning of this chapter, each psychological and behavioural feature of an eating disorder will reinforce it, acting as a so-called maintenance mechanism. Strict dieting in particular is like adding fuel to the fire and acts through two main mechanisms:

1. *It works*. If dietary restraint successfully produces persistent undereating, losing weight is inevitable. In people with an eating disorder, the "buzz" or "high" they get from losing weight, combined with the symptoms of malnutrition, serves to reinforce their overvaluation. The outcome of this is not to stop extreme dieting, but instead to continue, and possibly even double down. Furthermore, not eating enough makes the problem even

worse, by causing so-called starvation symptoms, which themselves feed into the eating disorder, as detailed in the next section.

2. *It is doomed to failure.* Unlike flexible dietary guidelines, extreme, inflexible dietary rules are tremendously difficult to stick to for any length of time. As such, extreme dieting is likely to lead to binge eating (whether objective or subjective). People who overvalue their shape, weight or control over eating react badly when they break a dietary rule (even though the biological drive to eat made this almost inevitable), and at this point some will temporarily "give up" their rules and binge. As explained earlier, an objective or subjective binge-eating episode triggers feelings of guilt and shame, compounding the desire to diet to excess (and/or practice other compensatory behaviours) in order to "make up" for the binge.

Fast Fact

Despite the negative consequences of strict dieting, most people with eating disorders see dietary rules not as a problem but rather as a measure of their strength and willpower. They are an expression of their identity as "good dieters." If they see themselves failing at dieting, they believe that it is because they are weak, rather than because their dietary rules are too rigid and extreme. In those who binge eat, extreme dieting is generally one of the main means they use to compensate for a binge-eating episode, while those who have been or are overweight see this type of dieting as perfectly reasonable.

Low weight and starvation symptoms

Before losing weight, I was a really cheerful person. I had lots of friends and was always happy to spend time with them. I am a completely different person now. I think about food all day long. I am irritable and depressed and have no interest in going out with my friends. I am always cold and tired and can only manage to sleep a couple of hours a night.

Low weight and undereating cause serious physical complications and dramatic personality changes. It has negative repercussions on a person's way of thinking, emotional state and interpersonal relationships. This is the so-called *starvation syndrome*, which we know all about thanks to a ground-breaking experiment carried out at the University of Minnesota in 1944 and 1945. This we now know as the Minnesota Starvation Experiment, and it provided invaluable information on the behavioural, psychological, social and physical effects of low body weight and undereating. The following paragraphs summarise what the research team did, and what they found out.

The Minnesota Starvation Experiment and the effects of semi-starvation

The Minnesota research team (led by Dr Ancel Keys) wanted to study how a lack of food affects people in order to help famine victims in Europe and Asia during and after World War II. They recruited 36 fit, healthy, young, male conscientious objectors and subjected them to:

Phase 1 A 12-week control period in which the volunteers ate normally, with no calorie deficit (average daily energy intake around 3,492 calories)
Phase 2 24 weeks of semi-starvation (around 1,570 calories per day)
Phase 3 12 weeks of refeeding

Four of the volunteers dropped out either during or at the end of the semi-starvation phase, so most of the results reported were observed in 32 men only. Although individual responses to weight loss varied considerably, all the men experienced dramatic physical, behavioural, psychological and social changes, which are summarised next. Following is an overview of the effects of semi-starvation, and what these observations tell us about the effects of low weight and undereating in people with an eating disorder.

Physical

All the men lost approximately 25% of their body weight during the 24 weeks of semi-starvation. They experienced dramatic physical effects, including: vague abdominal pain, slow and difficult digestion, sleep disturbances, dizziness, headaches, hypersensitivity to light and noise, reduced strength, oedema (swelling caused by excess fluid trapped in the body's tissues), hair loss, decreased tolerance to cold (cold hands and feet), vision disorders (spots in the visual field and difficulty focusing on images). There was also a reduction in their resting body temperature and energy consumption, and both their pulse and breathing rates slowed. ➧ *These are the same physical symptoms reported by people with an eating disorder who are undereating and low weight.*

Psychological

The men experienced great cognitive and emotional changes. Their thinking appeared to become inflexible, and they had significant difficulty switching from one topic to another. They found decision-making difficult and tended to procrastinate. Although there were no changes in their IQ, there was a big drop in their ability to concentrate (likely due to recurrent distracting thoughts about food and eating), as well as their insight and critical judgement. All of them experienced mood changes, with some becoming depressed and others swinging between bouts of euphoria and depression. Many showed frequent signs of irritability and outbursts of anger, as well as an increase in general anxiety. The very fact that they are not eating enough causes massive changes in their personality. *These are the same psychological symptoms reported by people with an eating disorder who are undereating and low weight.*

Behavioural

The Minnesota men began to behave very strangely during the semi-starvation phase. Their eating became like a sort of ritual, governed by peculiar rules like only eating alone, eating food items in a fixed order, only from one particular plate at a specific seat, or wearing certain clothes. Some spent two hours eating a meal, eating very slowly, chewing every mouthful a fixed number of times and/or cutting food into small pieces or shapes. Their routines tended to become inflexible and rigid, and they often experienced difficulties in being spontaneous. Some exercised excessively, while others became lethargic. *These same behavioural symptoms are seen in people with an eating disorder who are undereating and low weight.*

Social

Being low weight and undereating can have a dramatic effect on social functioning. People tend to become inward-looking and self-focused, which leads to social withdrawal. They are less interested in spending time with friends or doing the things that used to give them pleasure. The hormonal disruption caused by weight loss is also accompanied by a marked decrease in sexual interest, masturbation and erotic fantasies. *The social effects of semi-starvation observed in the Minnesota Experiment are also the same as those reported by people with an eating disorder who are undereating and low weight.*

What does the Minnesota Starvation Experiment tell us about eating disorders?

The main piece of information we get from the experiment is that there is such a thing as *starvation syndrome*. This means we can distinguish between the symptoms that are specific to an eating disorder like anorexia nervosa and those that are the consequences of being underweight. This is important because if a symptom is merely a physical, psychological, behavioural or social effect of malnutrition, the only way to cure it is a healthy diet. This explains why an essential part of the treatment of eating disorders is to normalise body weight.

These "starvation symptoms" are summarised in Table 3.1. They are those symptoms that are not integral to an eating disorder but rather are

Table 3.1 The symptoms of starvation

Physical effects

- Loss of menstruation
- Abdominal pain
- Slow, difficult and uncomfortable digestion
- Sleep disturbances
- Dizziness
- Headache
- Weakness
- Hypersensitivity to light and noises
- Swelling (due to a build-up of fluid in the body)
- Cold intolerance
- Abnormal skin sensations (tingling, pricking, chilling, burning, numbness with no apparent physical cause)

Behavioural effects

- Increased mental rigidity and loss of spontaneity
- Eating rituals (eating very slowly, cutting food into small pieces, mixing food in a bizarre way, eating very hot spicy food)
- Spending a lot of time reading cookbooks and collecting recipes
- Increased interest in food that leads, for example, to visiting supermarkets
- Hoarding food
- Hoarding objects
- Drinking a lot of coffee and/or tea
- Increasing the use of salt, spices, chewing gum, hot soup and/or water
- Nail-biting
- Smoking more
- Binge-eating episodes
- Self-harm

Psychological effects

- Inflexible thinking
- Procrastination
- Poor concentration
- Poor insight and critical judgement
- Preoccupation with food and eating
- Depression
- Mood swings
- Irritation
- Hunger
- Anxiety
- Apathy
- Psychotic episodes
- Personality changes

Social effects

- Social withdrawal
- Loss of sexual desire

consequences of low weight and undereating. They are not the foundations of the illness but do contribute to maintaining it.

FOR THE SCIENCE:

Keys, A., Brozek, J., Henschel, A., Mickelsen, O., & Taylor, H. (1950). *The biology of human starvation*. Minneapolis, MN: University of Minnesota Press.

As seen in the Minnesota Experiment participants, food deprivation usually triggers severe preoccupation with food. It can lead some people to read cookbooks obsessively, talk about food incessantly, collect recipes, spend a lot of time in the kitchen, visit supermarkets unnecessarily, open and close food cupboards without eating, watch cooking shows and cook for others and/or feed others. Others hoard food, objects related to food or even objects unrelated to food.

While some people can tolerate hunger, for others it can become unbearable, and, as a result of their preoccupation with food, can eventually lead to binge-eating episodes, followed by intense distress. Some get hyperactive to burn as many calories as possible, but when the malnutrition is severe, they eventually become tired, weak, inattentive and apathetic and complain of lack of energy.

In other words, in addition to drastically reducing your quality of life by themselves, in one way or another, undereating and being low weight serve to reinforce or maintain your eating disorder. For example, the heightened sense of fullness and constant preoccupation with food and eating that come as a side-effect of low weight and undereating make any increase in food intake difficult. As explained earlier, starvation symptoms also maintain the overvaluation of shape and weight. For example, social withdrawal makes it difficult or impossible to develop other self-evaluation domains. Since such people have few other interests to take their mind off their shape and weight, their preoccupation with body image also tends to increase, thereby "cementing" the house of cards in place.

For these reasons, a vital part of treatment is to help people with eating disorders understand that low weight and undereating are problems in their own right. Starvation symptoms are inevitable consequences of malnutrition, and these not only affect your physical health but also extend to all areas of your psychological and social functioning. The men in the Minnesota Experiment suffered from these symptoms, despite not having an eating disorder. As soon as they returned to a healthy weight, these starvation symptoms gradually disappeared, and they were able to resume life as normal. Although the psychology underlying the eating disorder will also need to be addressed, in order to restore normal behaviour and set your real personality free, it is essential to eliminate the starvation symptoms that reinforce it. The only way to do this is to establish a pattern of regular eating and normal body weight—a fundamental goal of CBT-E.

Binge-eating episodes

> *Even if I am not physically hungry, I suddenly get a strong urge to eat. I start to gobble down large amounts of food very fast, and I can't stop until I am bursting at the seams. Initially, I feel quite high, but I quickly become terrified of gaining weight, and I feel so depressed and guilty about myself afterwards. I have no willpower.*

Binge-eating episodes are common in people with eating disorders. They are reported by about one-third of people with anorexia nervosa and everyone who is diagnosed bulimia nervosa and binge-eating disorder. There are two types of binge-eating episodes:

1. *Objective binge-eating episodes* are characterised by the intake of a large amount of food over a discrete period of time and associated with a sense of loss of control (e.g., a feeling that you cannot stop or control what and how much you are eating). There is a wide range in the amount eaten per episode, but it is typically between 1,000 and 2,000 kcal. For most people who binge eat, excluding those with binge-eating disorder, the objective binge-eating episodes occur in the context of severe dietary restraint (see earlier).
2. *Subjective binge-eating episodes* are also characterised by a sense of lack of control. However, the amount actually eaten during these episodes is not large, even though the individual perceives the amount eaten as being too much or excessive. This binge-eating episode, which may or may not be followed by purging, is common in underweight young persons and can be just as distressing and impairing as objective binge-eating.

Objective and subjective binge-eating episodes are not mutually exclusive, meaning that a person with an eating disorder may do both.

Why is binge eating so bad?

In short, it has major unfavourable effects and it maintains the eating disorder. The first moments after a binge are often pleasant; negative emotions are calmed, and hunger and a sense of deprivation disappear. However, these positive effects do not last long and are quickly replaced by disgust, guilt, self-loathing and depression. The fear of gaining weight quickly grows, and this can be so strong that it prompts compensatory behaviours (self-induced vomiting, misuse of laxatives, fasting, excessive exercise). In severe cases, all aspects of life are affected: work, relationships with friends and family and childcare. The most common long-term negative consequences of binge-eating episodes are the following:

- Damaged interpersonal relationships
- Worsening quality of life
- Depression
- Self-loathing
- Despair
- Social anxiety
- Irritability and anger
- Self-harm

Binge-eating episodes maintain the eating disorder through the following main processes:

- They increase concerns about shape and weight.
- They intensify dieting to compensate for the calories consumed during the binges.
- They may prompt the use of compensatory behaviours (e.g., self-induced vomiting, laxative misuse).
- They are used as a dysfunctional coping strategy for stressful events and aversive mood changes.

Is binge eating a form of addiction?

Although there are some similarities between binge eating and addiction, like cravings and urges, feelings of loss of control and use of the behaviour as a coping mechanism, there are essential differences. These can be summarised as the following points:

- *People who binge eat do not target specific classes of foods.* If binge-eating episodes were a form of addiction, they would be characterised by the desire for certain foods. The distinctive aspect of binge-eating episodes is the amount of food taken in, not the type of food eaten.
- *People who binge eat have a continuous urge to not to do so.* They do not want to do it, and only when they lose control do they succumb. In contrast, people with a **substance use disorder** are driven by the urge to smoke, drink or inject their poison. The last thing they want to do is stop.

> JARGON BUSTER
>
> **substance use disorder (SUD)**: the technical term for addiction. It arises when a person continues to drink alcohol or use another drug despite the fact that it causes problems with their health, relationships and daily life.

- *People who binge often do so after adopting a strict diet to lose weight.* Their aim is to practice the opposite behaviour, but, as we have seen, dieting increases their vulnerability to binge-eating episodes. To get hooked on a drug, however, you need to try it first, not avoid it.
- *People with binge eating often overvalue shape and weight.* Most people with bulimia nervosa and about half of people with binge-eating disorder report the overvaluation of shape and weight. They judge their self-worth almost exclusively in terms of their weight, shape and ability to control them. While overvaluation plays an important role in maintaining eating disorders and binge eating, it is not a characteristic of people with substance use disorder.
- *There is no direct relationship between binge eating and substance misuse.* The rate of substance and alcohol misuse in people who binge is higher than in the general population, but similar rates of addiction are seen in people with other mental disorders. Likewise, the rate of binge-eating is higher in people who abuse alcohol or drugs, but no higher than in individuals with other mental disorders. Even growing up in a family where drug abuse is rife does not make it any more likely that a person will binge eat than develop another mental disorder.
- *Those who stop binge eating do not start drinking excessively.* Although eating disorders have been observed to **precede** alcohol abuse (i.e., they arise at an earlier age), data on treatment indicate that those who stop binge eating do not replace the behaviour with alcohol abuse.

JARGON BUSTER

precede (verb): occur before

FOR THE SCIENCE:

Dalle Grave, R. (2021). Why binge eating may not be a form of addiction: A theory of poor validity and clinical utility. *Psychology Today*. Retrieved from www.psychologytoday.com/intl/node/1166429/preview

Excessive exercising

> *It is almost impossible for me to sit and relax. I stand up and walk when I can, even if I am exhausted or have no real place to go. I also try to do 300 push-ups and 500 sit-ups every day.*

Excessive exercising is a common feature in young people with an eating disorder, particularly those of low weight, and in some people it even precedes dieting. We consider exercising to be excessive when it is done too often, too hard and/or for too long, beyond that required for physical health. This is not the same as the training that an elite athlete does before a marathon, say, which may be given temporary priority but does not become the "prime directive."

There are three major forms excessive exercising generally takes on, including:

1. *Exercising too often*, like going to the gym twice a day
2. *Exercising too much*, for example doing excessive numbers of reps, push-ups or sit-ups
3. *Extreme daily activity*, such as standing and pacing rather than sitting down, and walking excessive distances

People with an eating disorder who exercise excessively feel a sense of being driven or compelled to do so, and guilt and anxiety when they don't. Not only does excessive exercise increase the risk of physical injury, it also takes time away from other activities (e.g., school or work). When you ask people who exercise excessively why they do it, they generally give one or both of the following reasons:

- *To control shape and weight.* This is the most common function of exercise adopted by people with an eating disorder. Like extreme dieting, it can be compensatory (to make up for something) or non-compensatory. Sometimes compensatory exercising may be tactical, with people seeking to burn off calories before they actually ingest them (so-called debiting). Some feel that they can only eat if they have exercised beforehand, while other compensatory exercisers may adjust their physical activity levels in line with what they have already eaten.
- *To modulate mood.* Although less common, excessive exercising may also be used by some people for the high, or to block out or distract from aversive emotional states. In other words, they do it to make themselves feel better.

Exercising can't really be all that bad for you, can it?

Of course, a moderate amount of physical activity is necessary for good health, but exercise can actually damage your health when it becomes excessive. Excessive exercising has several negative consequences, affecting every sphere of a person's life, for example:

- It increases the risk of minor injuries such as repetitive strain, bone fractures and dislocations.

- It may have life-threatening consequences such as heart attack.
- It takes up a lot of time and **marginalises** other important activities and personal relationships.
- It requires secrecy and subterfuge and produces feelings of guilt.

JARGON BUSTER

marginalise (verb): think of or treat as insignificant

Like the other behavioural features mentioned previously, excessive exercising can maintain the eating disorder through several mechanisms:

- Alongside dietary restriction, it makes you lose weight and maintain low body weight, potentially leading to starvation syndrome.
- It increases hunger and therefore the risk of binge-eating episodes, a vicious cycle that may be established with both compensatory and non-compensatory exercising.
- It intensifies the overvaluation of shape, weight and their control. The more intensive and frequent the exercise to control shape and weight, the more time the individual spends worrying about their shape and weight, and vice versa.
- It leads to social isolation. Individuals with eating disorders typically exercise alone, and because they devote so much of their daily lives to it, they inevitably reduce the time they have to spend with others. The resulting marginalisation of their social life increases their loneliness and their overvaluation.
- It is a **dysfunctional** coping strategy. Although using excessive exercising to modulate mood may seem like a good idea in the short term, it is by no means a healthy way of dealing with problems in the long term. Learning to deal with unpleasant emotions should be a normal part of growing up, and there are functional ways to do this (your therapist will be able to help you). Think what would happen if you were suddenly unable to exercise. How would you cope then?

JARGON BUSTER

dysfunctional (adjective): not operating properly or normally

Self-induced vomiting

At first, it was a great relief to throw up. I thought I had found a simple method to make up for all the extra food I ate. But then I started bingeing more often, and now I spend all my days eating and throwing up. My stomach burns constantly, I have ruined my teeth, and my knuckles are really callused. The worst thing is that despite all this, I keep putting on weight.

Self-induced vomiting is practised by some young people with an eating disorder with the aim of reversing or minimising the effects of binge-eating episodes (objective and/or subjective) on weight. However, like excessive exercising, self-induced vomiting may also be used as a means of coping with upsetting events and associated mood changes.

At first, self-induced vomiting seems like an easy and effective method of weight control. But it is not a sustainable habit. Thinking they have a "get-out-of-jail free card," people who start this kind of purging tend to relax control of their diet, and their binge-eating episodes usually increase in frequency, leading to the need to vomit more often. People with long-lasting and/or frequent vomiting report feeling disgusted with themselves. They become self-critical because they think it is a "dishonest" means of controlling weight, when, as mentioned earlier and explained in the following section, it is not actually a means of controlling weight at all.

Does it actually work?

In a word: NO. A study on 17 women with bulimia nervosa conducted at the Human Nutrition of Pittsburgh found that *only a small part of the calories consumed during a binge-eating episode is present in self-induced vomit.* The study participants were asked to binge and throw up as they usually did at home, but the calorie content of both their binges and vomit were measured. Gross, we know, but a heroic effort in the name of science. Indeed, what they found was that no matter how much food they ate during a binge, a significant portion was left in the digestive system after vomiting. Whether they took in 3,500 kcal or half that, they retained over 1000.

> FOR THE SCIENCE:
>
> Kaye, W. H., Weltzin, T. E., Hsu, L. K. G., McConaha, C. W., & Bolton, B. (1993). Amount of calories retained after binge eating and vomiting. *American Journal of Psychiatry*, *150*, 969–971.

This finding explains why people with bulimia nervosa who use self-induced vomiting as a compensatory behaviour after binge-eating episodes seldom lose weight. Self-induced vomiting does not magically erase the calories you have, or the associated guilt; it only compounds the problem by creating a new vicious cycle.

But what can it hurt?

Self-induced vomiting has several negative consequences:

- *It is dangerous to your physical health.* Effects of self-induced vomiting range from the minor (callused fingers, enlargement of the salivary glands, erosion of dental enamel on the inner surface of the front teeth) to the potentially life-threatening (dehydration, low potassium in the blood and other **electrolyte** disturbances, which can lead to irregular heartbeat and even death).

- *It is dangerous to your psychological health*. It requires secrecy and deception and produces feelings of guilt and shame, potentially increasing levels of anxiety and depression.
- *It is dangerous to your social health*. Young people invariably feel the need to hide this behaviour and as a result often end up having to lie to the people they love. They also tend to avoid social occasions when food will be served, as they wouldn't be able to vomit afterwards.

> JARGON BUSTER
>
> **electrolyte** (noun): essential salts and minerals in the blood

Self-induced vomiting also makes it more likely that binge-eating episodes will continue, as people who do it think they have found an "out." However, as we have learned, it is impossible to throw up anything close to all the food that you take in.

Laxative and diuretics misuse

> *I tried to make myself sick after bingeing, but I just couldn't. I read somewhere that I could take laxatives to get rid of the calories from the food I ate. The number of pills I'm taking has gone up and up. I don't know why I keep gaining weight, because after taking laxatives, I feel cleaned out, like my stomach is empty. I am desperate.*

Once again, we are dealing with fake news. Thankfully, no one had to weigh poo to find this out, because only a basic knowledge of human biology was necessary to debunk the idea. Food is digested in the stomach and the small intestine. Laxatives empty the large intestine, which comes afterwards, and *absorbs only water and electrolytes, no food*. The "flat stomach effect," and any weight temporarily lost after taking laxatives, are only the results of watery diarrhoea. This will be reversed as soon as you eat or drink anything. Diuretics (aka water pills) also have absolutely no effect on calorie absorption. They can cause a temporary weight reduction by increasing urine output and therefore *reducing the body's water content*, until, of course, you have a drink. Once again, it is not calories that are being magically disappeared; it is only water.

Thankfully, the *misuse of laxatives and diuretics* is less common as a form of weight control than self-induced vomiting. However, some young people still haven't got the message and practice it either alone or in combination with self-induced vomiting. Like excessive exercising and other purging behaviours, laxative and diuretics misuse may be compensatory or non-compensatory. In other words, purging is used by some people in the doomed attempt to reverse the damage caused by a previous binge-eating episode (objective or subjective), whereas others use it as a "routine" form of weight control, not necessarily linked to episodes of overeating. Like binge eating, purging may also be used as a dysfunctional way of modulating mood.

What's the harm?

The misuse of laxatives and diuretics to control weight is not only ineffective but also dangerous. Aside from the obvious unpleasantness of watery diarrhoea, it is important to be aware that purging can be extremely harmful. To understand why, we need to return to biology class:

- The large intestine absorbs only water and electrolytes. Laxatives empty the large intestine, and therefore rid the body of water and electrolytes.
- Urine is made up water and electrolytes. Diuretics therefore eliminate water and electrolytes.

Thus, both laxatives and diuretics cause dehydration and electrolyte imbalances. This can be very dangerous and lead to heart attacks, among other severe, potentially life-threatening health conditions.

> FOR THE SCIENCE:
>
> https://medlineplus.gov/fluidandelectrolytebalance.html

Not only are laxatives and diuretics dangerous and ineffective, they also require secrecy and deception and produce feelings of guilt. Like bingeing and self-induced vomiting, their misuse needs to be hidden from loved ones. As above, this can lead to deception, social withdrawal and a sense of loneliness, making any underlying anxiety or depression worse. If used as a compensatory behaviour, laxatives and diuretics misuse maintains binge-eating episodes because, like self-induced vomiting, it is mistakenly seen as a "get-out-of-jail-free card." However, as we have seen, emptying the bowels or bladder is not the same as losing weight. In addition, using laxatives over a long period of time can lead to chronic constipation. This tends to create its own vicious cycle, increasing preoccupation with eating and stomach shape and perpetuating the perceived need to use more of these drugs, which, as well as being harmful, can become extremely expensive.

Fast Fact

Some young people with eating disorders manipulate their fluid intake to control their eating or weight. Typical abnormal drinking behaviours include drinking large amounts of water either to suppress the appetite and feel full or to make it easier to self-induce vomiting; repeatedly drinking and vomiting after a binge-eating episode until the liquid becomes clear of any food; and reducing fluid intake to dehydrate and "lose weight" (in reality, the loss of weight is due only to water). As explained in the biology lesson, altering the body hydration status can cause an electrolyte imbalance and potentially fatal consequences. Furthermore, all these behaviours maintain the eating-disorder mindset and make it more difficult to get well.

Other extreme weight-control behaviours

In addition to laxatives and water pills, other drugs such as appetite suppressants, thyroid hormones, cocaine and other substances are used for weight control by some young people with eating disorders, particularly those with binge-eating episodes. However, these drugs do not really produce significant and persistent weight loss. Appetite suppressants act only for a short period of time, and thyroid hormones mainly cause loss of muscle mass, not fat, for example. They all lead to serious physical complications and maintain the eating disorder, not to mention increasing the risk of developing a substance use disorder, too.

Some young people with eating disorders and type I diabetes reduce or omit their insulin dose after a binge-eating episode (objective or subjective). This insulin manipulation is not very effective at controlling weight, but can have devastating effects. It dramatically increases the blood sugar, causing ketoacidosis, coma and death. Even if it doesn't kill you, it increases the risk of severe diabetes complications in the long term, including cardiovascular disease, nerve damage and blindness.

Other unhealthy weight/eating-control behaviours practised by some people with eating disorders include excessive consumption of diet drinks, black coffee and/or sugar-free gums as appetite suppressants. The aim is to trick the body into feeling full, or to get the taste without taking in calories. These strategies are ineffective in the long term, and only serve to maintain the eating disorder. "Overdosing" on sweeteners and/or caffeine can also severely affect your physical health.

As we have seen, none of these extreme weight-control behaviours are effective, whether they are compensatory (i.e., after binge-eating) or non-compensatory (i.e., part of a non–binge-eating routine). All they do is reinforce the eating-disorder mindset by increasing overvaluation and the preoccupation with shape, weight and eating. In addition, many of them are extremely dangerous and habit-forming and may lead to life-threatening consequences or lifelong harm.

Body checking

> *I am entirely focused on controlling my weight. I weigh myself several times a day when I wake up, after meals, snacks and exercise. When I get up, the first thing I do is look at myself naked in the mirror. I look at myself for about five minutes, from the front, sides, and back, and pay special attention to how my belly, legs and behind look. I squeeze them to see how fat they are, and take a note of the change when I suck my belly in. I also look at my stomach in the mirror while I am dressing, and check how it looks when I'm dressed. I take photos and measurements of the body parts I don't like to keep track of any changes.*

It is very common for people to check their weight and body shape to some extent, but many young people with eating disorders display extreme forms of *body checking*. They check their body repeatedly, and often in an unusual way. Common examples of abnormal body checking include:

- Weighing yourself several times a day
- Examining particular body parts in the mirror (or reflective surfaces)
- Measuring body parts with a tape measure
- Pinching, squeezing or touching body parts, assessing the tightness of particular items of clothing (e.g., trouser waistbands) and accessories (e.g., watches or rings)
- Looking down at your thighs or stomach, for example, when sitting
- Taking photos of body parts on your phone
- Comparing yourself or your body parts with others' (including images on traditional and social media)

Generally, people with eating disorders examine their bodies with great attention to detail and for unusually long periods of time (scrutiny). They are extremely self-critical, and such checking can become so second nature that they may not be fully aware that they are doing it. For example, they may automatically compare themselves with others they see while walking down the street. When they do compare their bodies with others', they only tend to focus on the individuals whom they see as skinny and attractive (like models or actresses) or who have a particular physical feature they would like (for example a flat stomach). While they are overcritical of themselves, they look their chosen "role models" in a superficial and non-critical way. They do not compare themselves with people that are less skinny or attractive, so the outcome of these comparisons will always be the same: they are not thin, muscular or attractive enough.

How does body checking maintain eating disorders?

You probably know the drill by now, but body checking feeds into the eating-disorder mindset through the following mechanisms:

- Frequent weighing leads to misinterpreting tiny variations in body weight—generally due to a change in hydration status—as having gained weight. This encourages the intensification of dieting or the adoption of other extreme weight-control behaviours.
- You find what you look for. Repetitively scrutinising disliked parts of the body amplifies the perceived flaws and intensifies body dissatisfaction. This increases preoccupation with shape and weight and encourages more dietary restriction.
- Superficial and rapid observation of other people's body parts, especially if they are the perfect few, is like looking at them through a filter. You do not see the warts and wrinkles and therefore develop unrealistic ideas of what attractiveness is.
- Continually checking your body or comparing yourself with unattainable beauty standards can only reinforce the idea that your body shape is wrong, and therefore makes body dissatisfaction worse. Like the other psychological and behavioural features of eating disorders, both weight and shape checking form a feedback loop with overvaluation of shape and weight that needs to be disrupted.

Body avoidance

> *Since I started bingeing, I have completely stopped weighing myself, and I try to avoid leaving the house. I can't let my friends see me looking like this. If I have to go out, I wear baggy black clothes to conceal the shape of my ugly fat body.*

In the previous section, we saw that some young people with an eating disorder repeatedly check their body. At the other end of the spectrum are those who try to avoid looking at their bodies at all, and dislike having other people looking at them. This *body avoidance* may take on various forms:

- Avoiding weighing yourself
- Avoiding looking at yourself (e.g., not looking in the mirror, not having a bath and/or only getting dressed and undressed in the dark)

- Avoiding revealing your body shape (e.g., not wearing tight clothes and/or visiting places where the body is exposed, such as beaches, swimming pools and changing rooms)
- Avoiding certain clothing that may touch the body or feel tight (e.g., not wearing jeans or fitted clothes, but instead wearing loose, baggy clothing)
- Avoiding touching your own body (e.g., trying not to touch your body parts when washing)
- Avoiding being touched (e.g., not hugging or having intimate relationships)

Often these individuals have engaged in repeated body checking in the past but have switched over to body avoidance because their body checking became too distressing. Paradoxically, some people do both. For example, a person may check their belly in the mirror and then subsequently wear clothing that hides the shape of their stomach.

If I don't do it, how can it hurt me?

Body avoidance is problematic as it maintains the eating disorder through the following mechanisms:

- It allows concerns and fears about body weight and shape to persist without an objective reflection of what you actually look like. Your false beliefs about your body weight and shape remain unchallenged, and therefore do not have the opportunity to change.
- It rules out the possibility of receiving positive comments from others, and therefore your negative beliefs about your body are not called into question.
- It restricts interests, prevents intimate relationships, and leads you to isolate yourself, focusing even more on controlling your body shape and weight.
- Avoiding weighing maintains the fear of weight gain and facilitates weight gain or loss, as it prevents the use of measures to address the weight changes.
- Practising body avoidance is like sticking your head in the sand. The problem is that you don't see the tiger creeping hungrily towards you. If you already feel that you hate your body, ignoring it will only make that feeling worse.

Events, moods and eating

Events and emotions often influence people's eating behaviour. Some people comfort eat and some people lose their appetite when they are stressed or nervous, perhaps when they have a job interview or other life event coming up. Dietary changes associated with events and related mood changes are common in people with eating disorders and tend to be taken to the extreme.

As we have seen, some people use binge-eating episodes to distract themselves from problems that cause anxiety and to "dampen down" intense and intolerable emotional states. Other people use self-induced vomiting and/or excessive exercising to do the same thing. For example, if you feel nervous about an upcoming event, you might get the urge to eat uncontrolledly (binge eating) or less (dietary restriction), or even fast altogether. Alternatively, aversive emotions, mood swings and even certain events may make you want to exercise excessively, purge or practise some other dysfunctional coping mechanism.

Indeed, eating less, for example, might make you feel in control when you cannot control events or the emotions that they provoke, whereas overeating can be a way to achieve instant gratification. Eating less can also be a way to try to influence the behaviour of others. You might express feelings such as anguish or anger by refusing to eat. By harming yourself you might be (subconsciously or otherwise) trying to punish the people you love. This may not be true for you, but it is something we see often in underweight adolescents, who, for example, may stop eating in response to an argument with their parents.

Non-specific psychological features

Some people with eating disorders also have some coexisting pronounced psychological problems that contribute to the maintenance of their illness and interfere with treatment. We call these problems *non-specific* as they can also be observed in people with other psychological disorders. The most common non-specific factors maintaining eating disorders are described in the following sections.

Clinical perfectionism

As we saw above, people with an eating disorder are dissatisfied with their bodies and always striving towards that "perfect" thin or muscular ideal. It should come as no surprise then to learn that they often display perfectionist traits. Naturally, exacting standards are not necessarily a bad thing, but sometimes they can be so extreme that they interfere with the quality of a person's life and so rise to the level of *clinical* perfectionism.

The key feature of clinical perfectionism is a dysfunctional self-evaluation system. Such individuals judge themselves only or mainly on their ability to meet extremely high and demanding self-imposed standards in at least one important life domain, like school, sports or relationships. They want to be the best and are not concerned about the consequences on other areas of their life—the only thing that matters is reaching their goal. This *overvaluation of achieving* is similar to the overvaluation of shape, weight, eating and their control. Both are dysfunctional, fragile and unstable ways of judging yourself.

Clinical perfectionism has various harmful expressions that maintain the overvaluation of achieving. For one, it encourages *performance checking and/or avoidance* (like the body checking and avoidance discussed previously). This can result in over-scrutiny or procrastination and is driven and fuelled by the underlying feeling of never being good enough. Indeed, even when such people manage to meet their demanding standards, the first thing they do is to reset the bar: they set an even higher goal to achieve. Thus, there is no satisfaction to be had, no sense of achievement, which is precisely the feeling they are aiming towards. Obviously, such hyper-focus on performance leads to marginalisation of other areas of life and social withdrawal.

It is not yet clear to what extent perfectionist traits can interfere with eating-disorder treatment, but there is no doubt that *clinical perfectionism* makes people extremely unhappy. When clinical perfectionism coexists with eating disorders, there is an interaction between both problems. Perfectionist standards can become focused on achieving flawless control of shape, weight and eating. In other words, clinical perfectionism intensifies aspects of the eating disorder, like dietary restriction or excessive exercising. This complicates the treatment, and so if you have clinical perfectionism, it is crucial to tackle it head on. With this in mind, the broad form of CBT-E has a special module designed to treat clinical perfectionism along with the eating disorder.

Core low self-esteem

Most people with an eating disorder have low self-esteem. They are highly critical of themselves because they are not able to achieve their shape, weight and eating-control goals. We call this form of negative self-evaluation *secondary self-criticism*, because the primary cause is the eating disorder. This means that this aspect of their negative self-evaluation does not need any specific treatment, because it generally does not interfere with treatment and improves spontaneously once the eating disorder is in remission.

Some people, however, have underlying, or primary, extremely low self-esteem. They have an unconditional and pervasive poor opinion of their self-worth. Because this is long-lasting and does not seem to depend on circumstances or performance, we call this *core low self-esteem*.

People with core low self-esteem believe that they have little or no value, and describe themselves as "worthless," "useless," "stupid," "unlovable," and/or "a failure." They also tend to make unfavourable comparisons with others ("She/he/everyone is so much better/thinner/more intelligent than I am").

Other specific features of core low self-esteem are pessimism—an extremely negative view of the future; and hopelessness—the belief that positive change is impossible. We call these attitudes "negative cognitive biases," which tend to undermine the treatment.

When core low self-esteem coexists with the eating disorder, it obstructs positive change through two main processes:

1. Affected individuals see little or no prospect of recovery because of the unconditional and pervasive nature of their negative view of themselves.
2. The presence of core low self-esteem leads people to strive especially hard to control their shape, weight and eating to improve their sense of worthlessness.

With core low self-esteem, the chances of treatment success are poor unless low self-esteem is directly addressed. The broad form of CBT-E includes a special module with specific procedures to tackle it and improve it.

Marked interpersonal difficulties

Interpersonal difficulties—another way of saying problems with relationships—are common in people with eating disorders. As we have seen, some typical eating-disorder behaviours encourage secrecy and withdrawal from society. If these problems are secondary to the eating disorder, they generally don't interfere with treatment progress and often resolve spontaneously when the eating disorder goes into remission. For this reason, they do not need to be directly addressed by CBT-E. However, some people have severe, or marked, difficulties interacting with people before the eating disorder onset. These primary interpersonal difficulties act to feed into their eating disorder and/or make treatment difficult to undertake. Some examples of marked interpersonal difficulties that tend to maintain the eating disorder and/or interfere with the implementation of the treatment are described in the following paragraphs.

- *Social isolation and interpersonal-functioning deficit.* The most frequent interpersonal problem in young people with eating disorders is a lack of fulfilling relationships. People with this problem have poor social skills, struggle to meet and connect with their peers or react strangely to relationships. In these situations, pursuing thinness can become a dysfunctional way of trying to please others and develop more intimate and satisfying relationships.
- *Interpersonal conflicts.* These typically occur when a person and at least one significant other do not share the same expectations about the roles they should have in the relationship. Arguments of this nature may be present with any important figure in the life of a young person with an eating disorder, including parents, siblings and friends. Interpersonal conflicts can trigger and maintain eating disorders in some individuals. In an example case, one of our patients, a 17-year-old girl, was constantly treated like a child by her mother, while she would have liked to be more independent and autonomous. The girl controlled her eating to assert her independence

and autonomy towards her mother, who unfortunately reacted by treating her daughter even more like a child. In another case, a teenager used binge eating to regulate the negative emotions triggered by a conflictual relationship with his father.
- *Dealing with puberty and role transition.* It is not easy to be a teenager. This age group must deal with significant changes in hormone levels, body shape, environment (e.g., starting a new school) and roles ("growing up"), which may be confusing and distressing. Puberty begins in early adolescence, and the resulting development of *secondary sexual characteristics* (i.e., pubic hair, breasts and changing hip shape in females and increased muscle mass in males) can trigger anxiety and vulnerability in some teens. They feel destabilised by these changes and want to return their known and "safe" childlike bodies. Adolescence is also a period in which some experiment sexually for the first time. Indeed, their changing bodies attract greater attention (like wolf-whistles, cat-calls and compliments), which some may find difficult to handle.

Marked interpersonal difficulties can maintain the eating disorder through several mechanisms:

- They intensify the overvaluation of shape, weight, eating and their control, as they hinder the development of other self-evaluation domains.
- They can drive an individual deeper into their eating disorder to escape, avoid and distract themselves from their interpersonal difficulties.
- They may worsen self-esteem and encourage the use of shape, weight and eating control to improve self-evaluation.
- They may trigger episodes of binge eating, and there is evidence that patients with bulimia nervosa tend to be particularly sensitive to social interactions.

Mood intolerance

Events and emotions influence the eating of almost everyone, including those with eating disorders (see above). However, in some young people with eating disorders, eating is **markedly** influenced by events and associated mood changes. These people suffer from a problem called *mood intolerance*, which is characterised by two principal components:

> JARGON BUSTER
>
> **markedly** (adverb): significantly, to a noticeable extent

1. Extreme sensitivity to intense (especially aversive) mood states, and an inability to accept and deal appropriately with them.
2. The use of dysfunctional mood modulation behaviours to reduce the intensity of and neutralise negative emotions comes at a personal cost.

In people without an eating disorder, dysfunctional mood modulation behaviours may involve self-harming (for example, cutting or burning the skin) and/or taking psychoactive substances (for example, alcohol or other drugs). In people with both mood intolerance and an eating disorder, however, these problems are multiplied. They often discover that some characteristic eating-disorder behaviours, like binge eating, self-induced vomiting and excessive exercising, can be used as dysfunctional coping mechanisms: they help them deal with their negative emotions and make them feel better in the short term. In these cases, mood intolerance needs to be addressed, as it maintains the eating disorder and is likely to interfere with treatment. This is why the broad form of CBT-E has a module specifically designed to treat mood intolerance.

Other general psychological problems

The transition from childhood to adulthood is a turbulent time, and a certain amount of confusion and discomfort is not out of the ordinary. However, if left untreated, an eating disorder can cause young people to suffer from severe psychosocial problems. At its worst, an eating disorder affects every aspect of life. It interferes with adjustment to puberty and "growing up" and prevents you mastering the skills necessary to becoming a healthy, functioning adult. We often see teens with an eating disorder that have either failed to develop psychologically or have even regressed to a state of complete dependence on their parents. This inability to develop age-appropriate relationships may extend to other social groups, and interpersonal interactions become severely compromised. This leads a young person becomes isolated, withdrawn and indifferent to most of the things that made them feel good at a time when families and peers are needed to support development. If the disorder persists until adulthood, the person's identity can be permanently damaged.

It is not only eating disorders, but also other issues with mental health that are on the rise. Feelings of *depression* are common among young people with eating disorders and can be severe. Although a low mood may be caused by undereating and/or binge eating, it is important for your therapist to find out whether or not this is true in your case. Real clinical depression, with persistent low mood, loss of psychological drive, uncharacteristic tearfulness, social withdrawal and thoughts of death and dying, will make it difficult for you to commit to an "active" treatment such as CBT-E. This may mean that you need to be prescribed antidepressants before you can start. Alternatively, your therapist may judge that your depression is actually a starvation symptom, and therefore you can be weaned off your depression meds as you progress through your eating-disorder treatment programme.

The same goes for *anxiety*, which is also common in people with an eating disorder, who can get especially anxious in situations that activate concerns about the control of eating, shape and weight. For example, some people with an eating disorder tend to avoid social occasions that involve social eating (e.g., a birthday party or a night out with friends) or some degree of body exposure (e.g., swimming, dancing, beach vacations). Dealing with, and learning to enjoy, such situations and other triggers for anxiety are all part of the CBT-E journey, so unless your therapist feels that it is interfering with your treatment, anxiety shouldn't be a barrier to overcoming your eating disorder.

Obsessional and compulsive features are very common in people with eating disorders, but especially so in young people who are low weight and undereat. Think of the food checking and body checking behaviours we learned about earlier, not to mention the strange ways that the men in the Minnesota Experiment handled their food. Doesn't that sound a little OCD to you? Once again though, it's a chicken or egg scenario—we just can't say which came first. What we do know, however, is that in many cases obsessive-type behaviours get worse at low body weights and better when weight is restored.

Other things that your assessing therapist will need to know about before deciding on the best course of treatment for you is any alcohol or drug use. In most countries they are legally bound to keep your secret, but in any case, it is important to 'fess up to them. Things you need to let them know about are your drinking habits, for example if you drink habitually or overdo it now and again, and any psychoactive substances you may take (whether legal or illegal). Only after you have discussed these things with your therapist will you be able to decide together if CBT-E is right for you.

In summary

All eating disorders share specific psychological and behavioural features. According to the transdiagnostic theory, the core feature is the overvaluation of shape, weight, eating and/or their control. Overvaluation directly or indirectly leads to all the other psychological (e.g., preoccupation with shape, weight and eating, fear of gaining weight, feeling fat) and behavioural (e.g., dieting, binge eating, other extreme weight-control behaviours) features of eating disorders. In turn, these psychological and behavioural features "maintain" the eating disorder by fuelling the overvaluation. CBT-E aims to break these vicious cycles.

Other characteristic psychological (e.g., preoccupation with eating, mood swings, irritability, rigidity, social withdrawal) and behavioural (e.g., rigidity, procrastination, eating slowly) manifestations of eating disorders appear to be the result of undereating and low weight. These will disappear upon refeeding and weight restoration during the CBT-E programme.

Some people with eating disorders have some pronounced coexisting non-specific psychological problems (e.g., clinical perfectionism, core low self-esteem, marked interpersonal difficulties and/or mood intolerance) that contribute to the maintenance of their illness and interfere with treatment. These need to be addressed during treatment, and CBT-E broad form has special modules for this purpose. Likewise, several general psychological problems (e.g., depression, anxiety, obsessive features) may coexist with the eating disorder but are often the consequence of low weight, undereating and the negative effect of the eating disorder on your life. These do not usually need to be treated directly, as they should lessen as CBT-E progresses.

• Take-home message

There is no way to get rid of an eating disorder without breaking the psychological and behavioural chains that bind you to it. This is precisely what CBT-E has been designed to do.

Further reading

Dalle Grave, R., & Calugi, S. (2020). *Cognitive behavioural therapy for adolescents with eating disorders*. New York: Guilford Press.

Dalle Grave, R., & el Khazen, C. (2022). *Cognitive behaviour therapy for eating disorders in young people: A parents' guide*. London: Routledge.

Fairburn, C. G. (2008). *Cognitive behavioural therapy and eating disorders*. New York: Guilford Press.

Fairburn, C. G. (2013). *Overcoming binge eating* (2nd ed.). New York: Guilford Press.

Garner, D. M. (1977). Psychoeducational principles in treatment. In D. M. Garner & P. Garfinkel (Eds.), *Handbook of treatment for eating disorders* (pp. 145–177). New York: Guilford Press.

Keys, A., Brozek, J., Henschel, A., Mickelsen, O., & Taylor, H. (1950). *The biology of human starvation*. Minneapolis, MN: University of Minnesota Press.

4

Physical features of eating disorders

The physical features typical of eating disorders are usually caused by a low-calorie diet, weight loss, purging behaviours and excessive exercising. Fortunately, therefore, most medical problems resulting from these behaviours are reversed through nutritional rehabilitation and weight restoration. This means that the management of most physical issues, albeit with a few exceptions, should mainly focus on reversing the eating disorder.

Physical effects of dieting and low weight

Maintaining a restrictive diet and being underweight have several adverse effects on your physical health. The nature and severity of those effects depend on the severity of the dietary restriction and the amount of weight lost. They also depend on your age. Adolescence is a time of great change in your body. This means that if your eating disorder is successfully treated early enough, some aspects of your health can "bounce back" with no lasting damage. However, precisely because your teen years are the time when your body develops, some physical complications will cause permanent damage. This is why you should seek treatment for your eating disorder as soon as possible. The following sections outline the health problems that typically arise in people with an eating disorder, providing an overview of what they are, what causes them, and how they can be treated or managed.

Fast Fact

A BMI below 18.5 kg/m^2 is considered underweight. BMI is calculated by dividing your body weight by your height squared.

BMI = your weight (kg)/your height (m)^2

DOI: 10.4324/9781003342489-5

Brittle bones

My eating disorder started at the age of 13 years. I went on an extreme diet, which led to progressive weight loss. Despite several specialised treatments and hospitalisations in eating-disorders units, I have always maintained a very low weight. Finally, at the age of 24, I restored my weight and accepted my natural body shape through cognitive behavioural therapy. Unfortunately, at the age of 30 years old, and despite my normal weight, I recently suffered a fracture of the thighbone. It turned out my bones had become brittle because of my years of being severely underweight.

> JARGON BUSTER
>
> **onset** (noun): when a disease starts

The **onset** of an eating disorder often coincides with the period of bone development, when young people have not yet reached peak bone mass, which usually occurs between 25 and 30 years of age. If adolescents with an eating disorder lose too much body weight, their bones don't develop properly (called osteopenia) and become brittle. The medical term for brittle bones is osteoporosis, which is more usually seen in elderly patients. However, if osteopenia occurs in teens, osteoporosis will arise much earlier. It will become permanent and increase the lifetime risk of fractures. Significant reductions in bone mass can usually be detected after six months of weight loss and are almost always present if BMI is lower than 15.0.

It is a common misconception that brittle bones are something that only affect females. This is not true. While in the general population osteoporosis is much more frequently seen in females, males with anorexia nervosa also may suffer from severe osteoporosis. Its severity depends on the duration of the eating disorder and the lowest weight reached—the longer the eating disorder and the lower the weight, the more severe the damage to the bones.

For females with anorexia nervosa, the cause of bone loss is multifactorial, that is to say, it depends on several things. As you know, when females lose too much weight, their period can stop (amenorrhoea). This is because their oestrogen levels get too low. Just like in women after the menopause, low oestrogen leads to increased bone resorption—the bone tissue is broken down and the minerals it contains, most importantly calcium, are carried away in the blood. So, low oestrogen is one cause of brittle bones, but that is not the only problem. Especially in teens, low weight and associated hormone changes actually affect bone formation. This means that any loss of bone is more severe than after menopause. Bone tissue is constantly being formed—a process called bone remodelling—and so to maintain a healthy, stable bone structure, as much bone needs to be formed as is lost. In post-menopausal women, it is usually healthy bone being degraded, while the bone loss in eating disorders is adding to the lack of healthy bone being formed—double trouble.

Fast Fact

Doctors can measure your bone density using low-dose X-rays. This is often called a DEXA scan, which you may be offered when you get assessed for treatment. Using the DEXA scan, scientists have been able to measure the effects of weight restoration on bone density. They found that weight gain is an effective strategy for increasing bone mass in adolescents with anorexia nervosa, but that it can take some time. Typically, improvements do not become detectable until around 16 months of maintaining a normal body weight.

This combination of causative factors behind brittle bones explains why it cannot be treated by drugs alone. The high oestrogen doses given as an oral contraceptive do not improve bone mineral density. On the contrary, preliminary studies have shown that the physiologic transdermal oestradiol replacement (as used in menopause) increases spine and hip mineral body density in girls with anorexia nervosa who regain body weight. However, these results need to be replicated. To date, body weight restoration is the main valid and effective treatment of bone disease in anorexia nervosa.

FOR THE SCIENCE:

El Ghoch, M., Gatti, D., Calugi, S., Viapiana, O., Bazzani, P. V., & Dalle Grave, R. (2016). The association between weight gain/restoration and bone mineral density in adolescents with anorexia nervosa: A systematic review. *Nutrients*, *8*(12), 789. doi:10.3390/nu8120769

Fertility issues

Although no longer diagnostic, in females, amenorrhoea (when your period stops) is a key physical feature of eating disorders. Low weight, stress, weight loss and/or excessive exercising stop your body producing enough oestrogen to maintain your menstrual cycle. It is your body's way of saying that it is not a healthy enough environment to create and nurture a baby.

In fact, babies born to women with severe eating-disorder symptoms before pregnancy are born with a lower birthweight. This indicates that they are not receiving sufficient nutrition in the womb. There is also an increased rate of caesarean births in women with anorexia nervosa, not to mention a greater risk of unplanned pregnancy, presumably due to their irregular menstruation.

While oestrogen levels can be raised by taking the pill, as we learned in the previous section, this does nothing for bone health, and in any case, this would be like overriding the body's natural defence mechanism and tricking it into thinking that that it is healthy enough to bear a child. In addition, artificially restarting your periods could give you a false sense of normality and reduce your motivation to change.

Hence, weight restoration is the best treatment. While how much weight you need to regain to reverse secondary amenorrhea, i.e., loss of periods caused by an eating disorder, will vary from individual to individual, what is true for all is that accumulating some body fat is crucial for restarting the menstrual cycle.

FOR THE SCIENCE:

El Ghoch, M., Calugi, S., Chignola, E., Bazzani, P. V., & Dalle Grave, R. (2016). Body fat and menstrual resumption in adult females with anorexia nervosa: A 1-year longitudinal study. *Journal of Human Nutrition and Dietetics*, *29*(5), 662–666. doi:10.1111/jhn.12373

The good news is that once you regain the weight and your periods get back to normal, there will be no permanent damage. Females who wish to have children should not therefore be disheartened by the belief that their illness history will have caused irreparable fertility damage.

As for males, there is not much data available, but undereating and being underweight cause the male hormone testosterone to drop. As a consequence, they have a reduced sex drive and low sperm count and **viability**. Excessive exercising too can play a role, by keeping the testicles at a temperature too high for healthy sperm production. Furthermore, drugs taken to enhance musculature or reduce weight can play havoc with your hormones and, consequently, sexual function and development. Once again, drugs are not the answer, and only weight restoration as part of a treatment for eating disorders like CBT-E is the only sure-fire way to restore fertility.

JARGON BUSTER

viability (noun): ability to work or survive successfully

Brain damage

While no way near as severe as the damage caused by lack of oxygen or a traumatic brain injury, people who are malnourished and underweight often have altered brain structure and function. Studies indicate that individuals with anorexia nervosa have significantly less grey and white matter. This is because the brain is an organ that requires a considerable number of calories to function at its best.

Unsurprisingly, these structural alterations in the brain are linked with several psychological and social effects, as we saw in the men in the Minnesota Experiment (Chapter 3). However, the evidence suggests that if weight is restored in the early stage of the illness, this brain damage may be reversed.

FOR THE SCIENCE:

Walton, E., et al. (2022). Brain structure in acutely underweight and partially weight-restored individuals with anorexia nervosa—a coordinated analysis by the ENIGMA Eating Disorders Working Group. *Biological Psychiatry*, *9*(1), 730–738. doi:10.1016/j.biopsych.2022.04.022

Delayed or stunted growth

Malnourishment in teenagers, before the bones are fully developed, can cause growth to slow down or stop entirely. If undereating persists after 15–18 years in girls and 18–22 years in boys, they will be permanently shorter than they would normally be, because their bones have become stunted. However, if adolescents start regaining weight quickly, these growth problems are reversible.

Heart and circulatory damage

Extreme dieting and low weight can have a profound impact on your heart and blood vessels. Heart muscle is lost and becomes weaker with malnutrition and excessive weight loss. Blood pressure becomes low, as does the heart rate. Persistent low body weight also increases the risk of a dangerous alteration in heartbeat, especially if there is also a significant electrolyte imbalance due to self-induced vomiting and/or misuse of laxatives and diuretics. Once again, though, as they occur as a result of the eating disorder, these abnormalities completely resolve with proper treatment and weight restoration.

Digestive complaints

Dieting and weight loss are often associated with a persistent sense of hunger, although this may differ from person to person. An altered sense of taste may also be present, which explains why underweight people tend to use large amounts of spices to give flavour to the food they eat. If you don't eat enough, gut **motility** is slowed down, probably to maximise the absorption of food. Consequently, the food stays in the stomach for a long time before passing to the small intestine, giving the person a sense of fullness even after eating a small amount of food. Constipation is another frequent **gastrointestinal** symptom of patients with eating disorders and is also the result of reduced gut motility due to low weight and dietary restriction. Slowed gastrointestinal motility may also cause severe bloating.

> JARGON BUSTER
>
> **motility** (noun): ability to move

> JARGON BUSTER
>
> **gastrointestinal** (adjective): to do with the digestive system

In some cases, the misuse of laxatives may permanently damage the function of the intestine. However, all of the other digestive problems are easily reversed with nutritional rehabilitation and weight restoration. You may need to be hospitalised if you have a dangerous increase in liver enzymes, but our clinical experience tells us that these return quickly to normal level with rest, refeeding and weight regain.

Other common physical effects of dieting and being low weight

Malnourishment can affect every body system, as every body system needs energy to work properly. It stands to reason then, that if you don't provide your organs with the energy they need to do what they were built for, the systems will start to fail. Following is a brief overview of various problems that can arise with low body weight, all of which can be reversed if your weight goes back to normal.

- *Effects on muscles*. Undereating and low weight produce muscle loss, and weakness may result. When the person is severely underweight, there is a dramatic drop in fitness. This leads to their having difficulties walking up the stairs, squatting or standing up from sitting.
- *Effects on skin and hair*. A common consequence of being low weight is dry skin, which can develop painful cracks. The skin on the soles of the feet and palms of the hands may turn an orangey-yellow colour. Downy hair may sprout on parts of the body, particularly the arms, face, back and stomach. The extremities may turn blue due to a lack of oxygen in the blood. This most commonly occurs in the hands, although the feet and even parts of the face may be affected. Some experience hair loss from the scalp, and others have purple, brittle nails.

- *Body temperature*. A certain amount of body fat keeps you warm, and so your body temperature decreases if your body weight gets too low. A slowed metabolism due to malnutrition can also make you feel profoundly cold. To try and warm up, you may spend time sitting on radiators, having scalding baths or showers and/or wearing lots of layers.
- *Sleep disturbances*. Prolonged and severe dietary restriction produces insomnia and decreases the need for sleep, as we saw in the Minnesota Starvation Experiment (Chapter 2). Altered sleep patterns have also been observed in people with anorexia nervosa. These disturbances include reductions in total sleep time and quality and waking up several times a night. A study we conducted found that such disturbances are linked to body weight and the eating disorder's duration. In other words, the longer a person is affected, and the lower their body weight, the poorer the quality of their sleep. Once again, no drugs are needed to resolve these issues, which appear to clear up entirely once body weight is normalised.

FOR THE SCIENCE:

El Ghoch, M., Calugi, S., Bernabe, J., Pellegrini, M., Milanese, C., Chignola, E., & Dalle Grave, R. (2016). Sleep patterns before and after weight restoration in females with anorexia nervosa: A longitudinal controlled study. *European Eating Disorders Review*, *24*(5), 425–429. doi:10.1002/erv.2461

Physical effects of binge-eating

Effects on body weight

Binge-eating episodes may affect body weight, but the relationship is complex. When the binge-eating episodes start, people with bulimia nervosa and binge-eating disorder usually have normal body weight. However, while those with bulimia nervosa tend to maintain a normal weight, those with binge-eating disorder tend to gain weight. The reason depends on what the people eat between their binges and whether or not they use compensatory behaviours. The eating pattern of people with bulimia nervosa is characterised by an alternation of strict dieting, binge-eating episodes and compensatory behaviours. In contrast, people with binge-eating disorder tend to eat excessively and chaotically between the binges and do not rely on compensatory behaviours.

Binge eating usually has a minimal impact on the weight of people with anorexia nervosa, as their binges tend to be infrequent and subjective (i.e., not involve an objectively large amount of food). However, in about one-quarter of people with anorexia nervosa who binge eat, these episodes become progressively more frequent and involve increasingly large amounts of food. As a result, they start to put on weight, and their diagnosis may shift from anorexia nervosa to bulimia nervosa.

CBT-E is very effective at helping people stabilise their weight, whatever their diagnosis. It has strategies and procedures for stopping both binge-eating and dietary restraint. The result is a healthy diet and a balanced energy intake.

Effects on the stomach

The immediate effect of a binge-eating episode is a sense of fullness. In some cases, this sensation can become intense and painful. This effect is more intense in people with bulimia nervosa than in those with binge-eating disorder, probably because the former eat more quickly than the latter. Some people report that the sensation of fullness is accompanied by breathlessness. This may result from the **diaphragm** being compressed by the stomach, which has ballooned due to the large amounts of food ingested. On very rare occasions, people will eat so much that their stomach becomes massively enlarged, and may even burst. In this case, the pain is extreme, and there is a need for urgent medical intervention.

> JARGON BUSTER
>
> **diaphragm** (body part): the large muscle between the lungs and the stomach that helps you breathe

Physical effects of purging

Fluid and electrolyte alterations

We have already discussed how self-induced vomiting and/or misuse of laxatives and diuretics cause fluid and electrolyte imbalances. These alterations are very dangerous, especially if you take large amounts of laxatives and diuretics. They are also potentially life-threatening in those who try to "wash out" their stomach by repeatedly drinking fluids and vomiting until the vomit becomes completely clear. However, most of the vitamins and minerals our body needs to function correctly come from our food, and so if you are restricting your diet, the odds are you are not getting enough of them.

The most dangerous electrolyte alteration is low potassium. Our heart needs potassium to beat, and not having enough potassium in the blood can cause irregular heartbeat—a potentially life-threatening event. Low sodium may also be very dangerous, as it is necessary for blood circulation and nerve and muscle health. Sodium deficiency is usually due to purging, excessive water intake, undereating and/or or excessive exercising. Other electrolytes whose levels can become skewed due to dehydration include chloride, phosphate, magnesium and bicarbonate. Too much or too little of these electrolytes can cause severe medical complications. The main symptoms associated with electrolyte imbalance are extreme thirst, swelling of the legs and arms, weakness, muscle spasms and cramps and, in rare cases, epileptic seizures.

Your blood levels of these minerals and salts can be measured by a simple blood test, but to treat them you need to rehydrate and stop purging immediately. CBT-E can help you to do this.

Tooth damage

Repeated self-induced vomiting over a long period of time causes erosion of the tooth enamel, particularly to the inner surfaces of the teeth. As fillings are not damaged, as the enamel wears away, they will start to stick out. This erosion is irreversible, but will only stop once self-induced vomiting stops. There is no point treating such dental issues until their cause has been removed.

Other common physical effects of purging

SWELLING OF THE SALIVARY GLANDS

This is the consequence of frequent vomiting but—be warned—it can also arise if self-induced vomiting is stopped suddenly. The swelling, which mainly involves the parotid gland (the gland affected in mumps), is painless but makes you look a bit like a hamster with its cheeks full of nuts. Hence, sufferers often interpret this swelling as having a fat face and, consequently, a fat body. However, salivary gland swelling is reversible and goes away some time after stopping self-induced vomiting and normalising eating habits.

Damage to the oesophagus

In rare cases, violent self-induced vomiting can cause tears and bleeding in the **oesophagus** wall, and there is a slight risk of rupture. This damage urgently requires immediate medical intervention.

> JARGON BUSTER
>
> **oesophagus** (body part): the "food pipe" connecting your mouth to your stomach

Damage to the throat

Some people self-induce vomiting mechanically, using their hands or objects to stimulate their gag reflex. This forceful process can injure the back of the throat, which can become infected.

Damage to the hands

Individuals who use their fingers to stimulate their gag reflex usually develop bruised and scarred knuckles. This is due to the repeating rubbing of the knuckles on the teeth over time. This is known as "Russell's sign."

Fluid retention

Stopping laxatives and diuretics "cold turkey" after long periods of misuse may result in temporary weight gain. Although this will understandably increase preoccupation with weight, you shouldn't be tempted to start purging again, because this weight gain is due to water retention and is only temporary.

Physical effects of excessive exercising

Excessive exercise can negatively affect physical health. It leads to muscle pain, weakness and injuries, usually linked to increased creatine kinase in the blood. Creatine kinase is a protein found in your muscles and is released into the blood when they become damaged. Other injuries caused by excessive exercising include stress fractures—small cracks in the bone—or severe bruising within a bone. Most often these are seen in the toes, heel, lower leg and ankle, which can cause swelling and pain.

Clinical problems requiring prompt medical attention

All people with eating disorders, even if being treated by a psychologist and dietician, should be regularly assessed by a doctor who has good knowledge of the medical complications that may arise. The clinical problems associated with eating disorders that require prompt medical intervention are listed in Table 4.1. If you have or think you might have any of these, you must ask to see a doctor straight away.

Table 4.1 When to call the doctor

- Palpitations (when your heartbeat becomes more noticeable—your heart may feel like it is racing or beating very fast, pounding or fluttering and/or your heartbeat may be irregular, with skipped or extra beats)
- Severe fatigue
- Dizziness in a standing position or when standing up
- Feeling "light-headed"
- Chest pain
- Blood in vomit
- Mental confusion and/or memory loss
- Swelling (oedema) of the legs or arms
- Convulsions (uncontrollable muscle contractions)
- Self-harm
- Thinking about suicide
- Body mass index <15.0 kg/m^2
- Recent loss of more than 1 kg of body weight per week for two or more consecutive weeks
- Fasting or daily intake <500 kcal for two consecutive days or more
- Habitual and recurrent self-induced vomiting or other purging behaviours (misuse of laxatives and/or diuretics)
- Heart rate <40 beats per minute
- Low blood pressure
- Body temperature $<35°$ C

In summary

Medical complications in people with an eating disorder are the result of one or more of the following:

- Undereating
- Weight loss
- Dietary restriction
- Excessive exercising
- Purging

Although most of the physical effects of these factors disappear after weight normalisation, some complications, such as brittle bones, may cause permanent damage in young people.

• Take-home message

Most of the medical complications of an eating disorder are reversed with weight restoration and the adoption of healthy habits.

Further reading

Kimmel, M. C., Ferguson, E. H., Zerwas, S., Bulik, C. M., & Meltzer-Brody, S. (2016). Obstetric and gynecologic problems associated with eating disorders. *International Journal of Eating Disorders*, *49*(3), 260–275. doi:10.1002/eat.22483

Mehler, P. S., & Andersen, A. E. (2017). *Eating disorders: A guide to medical care and complications* (3rd ed.). Baltimore, MD: Johns Hopkins University Press.

Misra, M., Katzman, D., Miller, K. K., Mendes, N., Snelgrove, D., Russell, M., . . . Klibanski, A. (2011). Physiologic estrogen replacement increases bone density in adolescent girls with anorexia nervosa. *Journal of Bone and Mineral Research*, *26*(10), 2430–2438. doi:10.1002/jbmr.447

Robinson, P., & Rhys Jones, W. (2018). MARSIPAN: Management of really sick patients with anorexia nervosa. *BJPsych Advances*, *24*(1), 20–32. doi:10.1192/bja.2017.2

5

Is CBT-E right for me?

As we saw in the previous chapters, we don't know how or why people get an eating disorder, so they cannot yet be prevented. However, we have learned quite a lot about how the vicious cycle they put in motion works, and therefore how they can be treated.

While there is no drug, i.e., no medical treatment, there are good psychological treatments available. The evidence-based National Institute for Health and Clinical Excellence (NICE) guidelines, those looked to by healthcare professionals across the world, recommend enhanced cognitive behavioural therapy (CBT-E) for the treatment of all the forms of eating disorders in adults and young people. However, to understand if CBT-E is right for you, it is necessary to understand the theory they are based on.

CBT-E: the theory

Explaining why a person continues to adopt extreme weight-control behaviours to lose weight or maintain a condition of low weight, despite the adverse effects on physical health, psychological wellbeing and interpersonal relationships is a widely debated topic that has led to two very different explanations:

1. *The disease model.* According to this model, the characteristics of the eating disorder, such as strict dieting, fear of gaining weight and failure to recognise the severity of current low body weight, are the result of a specific illness, namely anorexia nervosa, bulimia nervosa or another eating disorder. The patients are considered not to be in control of their disease. Therefore, to overcome it they need external control by parents and/or healthcare professionals. Under this model, patients have a passive role in treatment—they are told what to do, and to get well all they have to do is follow instructions. This is the model upon which family therapy and medical treatments of eating disorders are based.
2. *The psychological model.* This is based on a psychological explanation of the patient's eating disorder; specifically, the young person has difficulties

DOI: 10.4324/9781003342489-6

seeing dieting and low weight as a problem because their self-evaluation scheme (how they judge themself) is mainly based on shape, weight, eating and their control. This explains why being able to diet and achieving a low weight is often associated with a sense of achievement, despite the negative consequences. According to this model, young people can be helped to understand how their eating disorder operates, and that their self-evaluation system is dysfunctional. Instead of being told what to do, they take an active role in their own treatment. Their therapist helps them develop functional solutions and implement changes to their mindset and behaviour. The aim is for them to rebalance and stabilise their self-evaluation scheme and, therefore, recover from the eating disorder. In other words, under this model, it is the patient, rather than the therapist or parents, who calls the shots. This is the model that CBT-E is built around.

As you may have guessed from the title of this book, we think that that the second option is the way to go. However, if at this point you think you would prefer to opt for family therapy or medical treatment for your eating disorder, this does not mean that you should put the book down now. Even if you feel that it is the therapist's job to "cure" you, rather than for you to take back control of your life from an eating disorder, you should read on. After all, knowledge is power, and the only good choice is an informed choice.

CBT-E: from theory to fact

The origins of CBT-E are in research in the early 1980s by Prof. Fairburn, whose team at Oxford was trying to understand and treat bulimia nervosa. They discovered that it was precisely these ways of thinking and behaving, along with their physical consequences, that reinforced or maintained the disorder. They identified several such vicious cycles or feedback loops operating in people with an eating disorder, whatever their actual diagnosis. They coined the term "maintenance mechanisms" to describe these feedback loops and concluded that all the main eating-disorder features stemmed from one "core" feature: the overvaluation of shape, weight and/or eating control.

They therefore designed a treatment to interrupt these feedback loops and thereby to lessen the overvaluation: cognitive behavioural therapy (CBT) for bulimia nervosa. CBT teaches you coping skills for dealing with problems. It focuses on how your thoughts, beliefs and attitudes affect your feelings and actions.

Given the success of cognitive behavioural therapy in bulimia nervosa, and indeed many other mental health conditions, Drs Fairburn, Cooper and Shafran took a look at how the theory applied to other eating disorders, and the transdiagnostic cognitive behavioural theory was born. In other words, these researchers found that the psychological and behavioural features, along with the associated maintenance mechanisms, seen in one eating disorder are often seen in another. To refresh your memory, the main psychological and behavioural features common to eating disorders are the following:

- Overvaluation of shape, weight and eating
- Preoccupation with shape, weight and eating
- Fear of gaining weight or getting fat
- Feeling fat
- Extreme dieting
- Binge-eating episodes
- Excessive exercising
- Self-induced vomiting
- Misuse of laxatives and/or diuretics (aka water pills)
- Body checking/avoidance

Fairburn, Cooper and Shafran also discovered that in a subgroup of people with eating disorders, there are four main types of psychological issues that appear to feed into the overvaluation. These psychological issues are clinical perfectionism, core low self-esteem, marked interpersonal difficulties and mood intolerance (discussed in detail in Chapter 3). These issues are not specific to eating disorders but do make them very difficult to treat. As not every person with an eating disorder suffers with these issues, they do not need to be treated in every case. Hence, there are now two types of CBT-E programme available: the "focused" form, which is designed to treat these main maintenance mechanisms, and the "broad" form, which contains additional modules to treat one or more of the non-specific features that are reinforcing it.

Since its inception, transdiagnostic cognitive behavioural theory has significantly contributed to what we know about eating disorders. The E in the CBT-E you may be offered today stands for "enhanced." Over the years, the effects of the original CBT-E have been studied in large groups of patients. This has taught us many valuable lessons, and we have refined and enhanced the treatment with these in mind. This means that the CBT-E that you can get today is the very best treatment that science has come up with, and there is no reason why it shouldn't work for you.

Main maintenance mechanisms

According to transdiagnostic cognitive behavioural theory, a distinctive self-evaluation scheme, mainly or entirely dictated by the *overvaluation of shape, weight, eating and their control*, is of central importance in maintaining eating disorders. Indeed, the other clinical features of eating disorders seem to arise either directly or indirectly from a person judging their self-worth in terms of their shape, weight and ability to control them. As we saw in Chapter 3, these include preoccupation with eating, weight and shape, feeling fat, various forms of body checking and/or avoidance and extreme weight-control behaviours (dietary restraint, dietary restriction, self-induced vomiting, laxative and diuretics misuse and excessive exercising). These features of eating disorders are expressions of the individual's belief that controlling their weight, shape and eating is of extreme importance in their self-evaluation.

The biological effect of undereating and other extreme weight-control behaviours is a persistent energy deficit. When weight becomes significantly low—as in most cases of eating disorders intercepted in young people—starvation symptoms develop. As discussed in Chapter 3, these starvation symptoms reinforce the overvaluation of shape and weight and **exacerbate** the undereating through the following maintenance mechanisms. These are mechanisms common to most people with an eating disorder, no matter their diagnosis:

> JARGON BUSTER
>
> **exacerbate** (verb): make worse

- The control of eating and weight achieved at the beginning of a diet makes you feel good and therefore intensifies your overvaluation of shape and weight.
- Undereating causes slow digestion. This means you feel full after even modest amounts of food. You may interpret this as having eaten too much and therefore increase dietary restriction.
- Undereating increases preoccupation with eating, which in turn may encourage you to adopt even stricter and more extreme dietary rules.
- The body reacts to dramatic weight loss by slowing the metabolism in order to stop you wasting away entirely. It essentially goes into survival mode and enables you to get by on very little energy. This means that you lose weight more slowly, which may prompt you to step up your efforts to restrict your diet or exercise excessively in order maintain a low weight and avoid weight regain.
- The social withdrawal that often occurs in people with an eating disorder isolates you from positive outside influences to distract you from or deter your overvaluation of eating, shape, weight and/or their control. You are essentially stewing in your shape, weight and/or eating concerns 24/7.

The one behaviour seen in many people with an eating disorder that is not a *direct* expression of the overvaluation of shape, weight, eating and their control is binge-eating. However, binge-eating does stem *indirectly* from overvaluation through the following mechanisms:

- *Undereating.* The overvaluation of shape, weight, eating and/or their control can prompt you to undereat. Doing so produces several changes in the hormonal and brain signals that control food intake. These signals tell you that you are hungry, encouraging you to eat more than you would otherwise. This is one of your body's natural defence mechanisms.

- *Extreme dietary rules.* Rigid dietary rules are impossible for most people to stick to long term, especially if they are also extreme. When they are broken, you may interpret this as evidence of your personal weakness and lack of self-control. As people with an eating disorder tend to have "all-or-nothing" thinking, they react extremely badly to such transgressions. Whereas being unable to resist temptation is not really a big deal for people without an eating disorder on a flexible diet, people who overvalue shape, weight and or eating control may essentially just give up their attempt to lose weight. This results in a binge-eating episode, which in turn fuels their concerns and beliefs about their lack of control when it comes to their shape, weight and eating. This leads to renewed or more extreme efforts at weight control, ultimately increasing the risk of later binge-eating episodes.
- *Events and associated mood changes.* These tend to maintain binge-eating episodes through three main mechanisms:

  1. When life difficulties and associated emotional changes inevitably occur, it gets even more difficult to stick to a restricted diet. This means that you are more likely to break your extreme dietary rules and therefore more likely to binge eat, as in the mechanism described earlier.
  2. Binge-eating temporarily improves mood and distracts from problems. It may become a dysfunctional means of coping with these difficulties.
  3. Binge-eating may be used for gratification or as a reward. Although this may seem strange, people with binge-eating episodes and obesity typically report this.

- *Self-induced vomiting or other compensatory behaviours.* These tend to maintain binge-eating episodes because of the false belief that such behaviours are effective in preventing calorie absorption. This removes a major deterrent to binge eating: the fear of gaining weight.

We can map all these interactions using a special flow chart called a "formulation." Figure 5.1 shows an example formulation describing the main specific maintenance processes operating in eating disorders. However, each person is different, and your own personal formulation will depend on your own beliefs and behaviour. For example, if you have been diagnosed with bulimia nervosa, your formulation will not contain the box "low weight and starvation symptoms" but may include all other eating-disorder features in the example formulation. If, on the other hand, your current diagnosis is anorexia nervosa, your formulation will definitely include the box "low weight and starvation symptoms," but maybe not the boxes "binge-eating" and/or "self-induced vomiting and/or misuse of laxatives." This type of formulation indicates the restricting type of anorexia nervosa. In the binge-eating/purging type of anorexia nervosa, as the name suggests, your formulation will include all three of these boxes. A young person with anorexia nervosa of the binge-eating–purging type will have the largest number of maintenance mechanisms in their formulation, while those with binge-eating disorder have the smallest number.

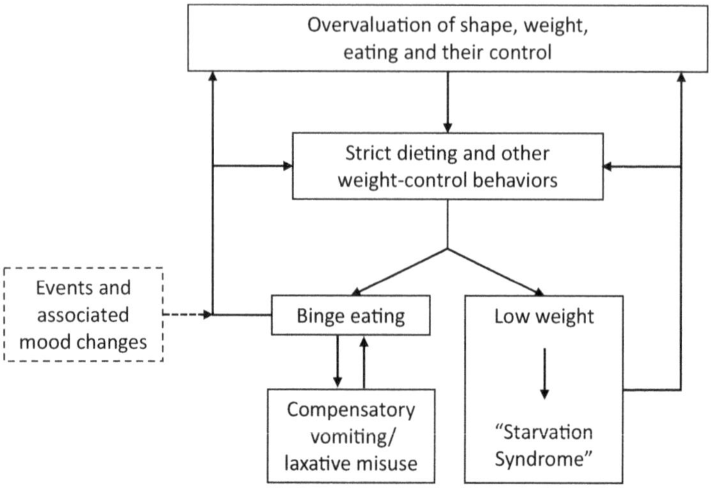

Figure 5.1 The processes involved in the maintenance of eating disorders, according to cognitive behavioural theory

Source: Adapted from Fairburn, C. G., Cooper, Z., & Shafran, R. (2003). Cognitive behaviour therapy for eating disorders: A "transdiagnostic" theory and treatment. *Behaviour Research and Therapy, 41*(5), 509–528. Copyright © 2003 Elsevier. Reprinted with permission.

The formulation is essentially a blueprint of your eating disorder as it is operating at the moment it is drawn up. It is a map of your individual manifestation of the eating-disorder features, and as such a guide to the processes that need to be tackled by treatment. The aim of CBT-E is to disrupt these mechanisms—to reduce the overvaluation by reducing the number of boxes feeding into it. Hence, the formulation represents an individualised road map to the focused form of CBT-E.

Non-specific maintenance mechanisms

According to cognitive behavioural theory, there are other psychological processes that may feed into the overvaluation and therefore need to be included in the formulation if present. These additional or "external" maintenance mechanisms are not specific to eating disorders and can make life difficult whether or not you have an eating disorder. However, when you do have an eating disorder, they act in a similar way to the main maintenance mechanisms described earlier. As they are non-specific, you may or may not have them. However, if one or more of them do apply to you, they are likely to make treatment difficult, and so they need to be tackled head on. This is what the "broad" form of CBT-E is for. Broad CBT-E is slightly longer than the focused form, as it contains extra modules designed to help you overcome:

- Clinical perfectionism
- Core low self-esteem
- Marked interpersonal difficulties
- Mood intolerance

These psychological issues, what they are and how they interact with the eating disorder are described in some detail in Chapter 3.

CBT-E: an overview

CBT-E is a psychological treatment based on the theory described earlier. It is suitable for all forms of eating disorders. The psychological model adopted by CBT-E explains why the treatment is collaborative and never asks you to do things you do not agree to.

For example, before you commit to starting treatment, you will be invited to attend a couple of preparation sessions. The point of these sessions is to give you the information you need to decide whether or not you want to give CBT-E a chance. As part of this process, the therapist will ask you to think about the pros and cons of starting the CBT-E. They will inform you that the goal of the first three to four weeks of treatment is not to make changes immediately, only to give you an opportunity to improve your understanding of the psychology behind your eating disorder maintenance mechanisms. This will put you in a better position to evaluate the implications of change. Even if your weight is low, you will not be asked to start restoring it straight away, only to decide that you would like to do so.

Once you have decided to start CBT-E, the focus will be to get you actively engaged in the treatment, to get you ready for change. To this end, you and your therapist will work together to understand your personal form of eating disorder, creating collaboratively a diagram or flowchart (in CBT-E terminology called "personal formulation") of the main processes that maintain your eating disorder, which will become the treatment's targets. You are also encouraged to observe how the processes in your personal formulation operate in real life. For this purpose, you will be asked to monitor specific aspects of your behaviour, thoughts and the associated feelings and events on a dedicated monitoring record. For example, you might be asked to write down what (a general idea, no weights and measures or calorie counting—the monitoring record is not a food diary) and when you eat, and any events, thoughts and feelings that influenced your eating. To be effective, this has to be done in real time, just after you eat, not at the end of the day.

Once you have a better understanding of the psychological and behavioural features that maintain your eating disorder, some sessions will be dedicated to evaluating the pros and cons of making the change. You will be encouraged to think about the way the eating disorder is affecting and will continue to affect your life. This should help you decide to tackle the features reported in your personal formulation, including weight regain if applicable. If you do not conclude that you have a problem to address, treatment cannot continue, but this seldom happens.

Then, if you agree to work on your issues, you will make some specific gradual changes to your eating and behaviour associated with your preoccupation with shape and weight. Once you have attempted this change, together with your therapist you will analyse what happened when you did and any effects it may have had on your way of thinking. Our patients usually find it much easier than they think to make these tiny changes, but if you do get into difficulties, your CBT-E therapist will teach you some problem-solving strategies to help you overcome them. This approach usually gradually reduces shape, weight and eating concerns and therefore helps you to get well.

Toward the end of the treatment, when your main maintenance processes have been disrupted, you will experience long intervals of time free from shape, weight and eating concerns. At this point the treatment shifts focus to helping you to recognise the early warning signs of a relapse. The aim is that by learning and applying CBT-E techniques, you will recover entirely from your eating disorder and never be bothered by it again.

The main goal

The main goal of CBT-E is to help you get well. This is achieved by helping you to make gradual changes to your thoughts and actions, shifting your self-evaluation scheme to one not mainly dictated by your shape, weight, eating and their control (Figure 5.2). When this has been achieved, you will be a healthier and happier person, and you should be able to get on with the rest of your life.

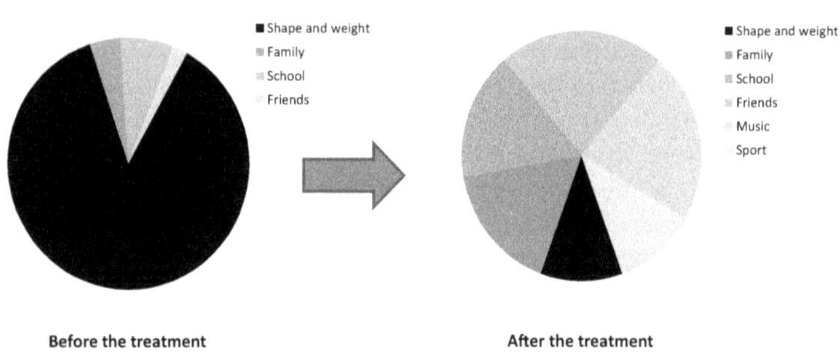

Figure 5.2 The main goal of CBT-E

Source: Reproduced with permission from *Cognitive Behaviour Therapy for Eating Disorders in Young People: A Parents' Guide* by Riccardo Dalle Grave & Carine el Khazen, Copyright © 2021 Taylor and Francis.

To achieve this goal, the treatment adopts the following general strategies:

- Actively engaging you in the treatment and decision to change
- Gradually removing the principal psychological and behavioural features of your eating disorder
- Correcting the mechanisms that maintain your eating disorder
- Making sure the changes are lasting

General structure

As you can see in Figure 5.3, after assessment and preparation, CBT-E for young people is delivered in three main steps, with regular review sessions. The steps are consecutive: each step adds something to the previous one. It is essential to start from the beginning and continue to the end, following the directions suggested by your therapist.

Assessment and Preparation

These two sessions will give you and your therapist time to get to know each other and for you to ask all the questions you need in order to make an informed decision about starting Step One of the treatment.

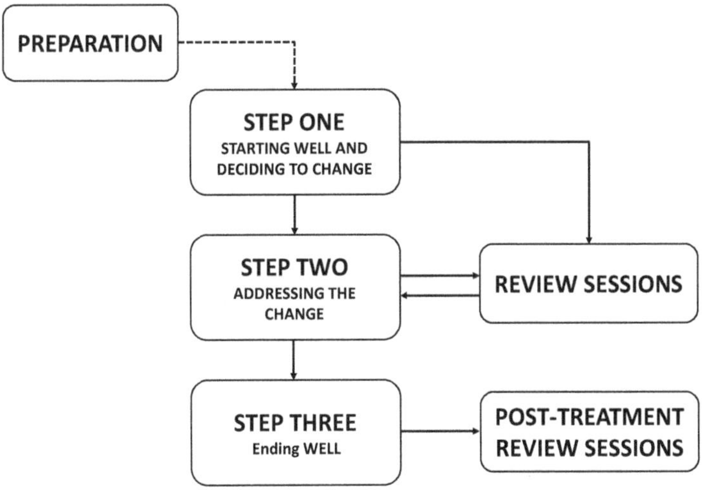

Figure 5.3 The CBT-E road map

Source: Reproduced with permission from *Cognitive Behaviour Therapy for Eating Disorders in Young People: A Parents' Guide* by Riccardo Dalle Grave & Carine el Khazen, Copyright © 2021 Taylor and Francis.

Step one—starting well

This step involves two sessions a week and lasts three to four weeks. During these sessions you will actively work with your therapist to achieve a shared understanding of the nature of your individual eating disorder and the main psychological and behavioural mechanisms that maintain it. You will start working on regularising eating (eating frequent meals and snacks, not changing the amount and type of food you eat at this stage) and reducing the frequency of your binge-eating episodes (if any). You will set up collaborative weighing with your therapist and learn to interpret any changes in your body weight. In this Step, if your weight is low, you will discuss with your therapist your reasons for and against attempting weight regain and change. Remember that in CBT-E, it is you who decides that you want to restore your body weight—no one will force you to do it. If you do not agree to work on regaining weight after four weeks, however, the treatment must be discontinued. At this point the therapist will help you find a treatment that is better suited to you.

Review sessions

In these sessions, you will talk about your progress with your therapist and make a plan for the coming weeks. They are also an opportunity to discuss with them any problems or doubts you may be having. Review sessions are scheduled at the end of Step One, and if you are low weight every four weeks during Step Two.

Step two—making the change

This is the main part of the treatment, in which you and your therapist will work to interrupt the main psychological and behavioural mechanisms that are maintaining your eating disorder. Usually, this involves addressing your concerns about weight and body shape, events and emotions that affect eating and dietary restraint. If you are underweight, you will also start weight regain strategies at the beginning of Step Two.

Step three—ending well

This is the final stage of treatment. At this point you will have regained control of your eating, and your behaviour will no longer be dictated by your eating disorder. The focus will now shift toward the future, with three fortnightly sessions dedicated to any concerns you may have about the end of treatment. The aim is to ensure the progress you are making is maintained and to help you minimise the risk of later relapse.

Post-treatment review sessions

You will be invited to check in with your therapist 4, 12 and 20 weeks after the end of the treatment. In these sessions you will discuss how things are going and how you have managed to cope with any remaining problems and setbacks.

The two forms of treatment

As we mentioned above, CBT-E can be administered in two forms:

1. *"Focused" form*. This only addresses the specific maintenance factors of your eating disorder. This is the form that we find is suitable for most young people, and it is the one described in this guide.
2. *"Broad" form*. This also has specific modules to help you overcome one or two of the following non-specific maintenance mechanisms:
   - Clinical perfectionism
   - Core low self-esteem
   - Marked interpersonal difficulties
   - Mood intolerance

The focused form is suitable for most young people. The broad form is reserved only for those whose non-specific maintenance mechanisms are pronounced, seem to maintain the eating disorder and interfere with their response to treatment. The decision to use the broad form of CBT-E is made collaboratively with your therapist in treatment review sessions.

How long does it take?

If you are not underweight, CBT-E generally involves two initial assessment/preparation sessions followed by about 20 individual sessions over 20 weeks. The treatment will be longer if you are underweight, usually taking 30–40 weeks. Each session lasts about 50 minutes each. In Step One the sessions are held twice a week so you can get some momentum going. Step Two sessions will be once a week if you are not underweight, but if you are underweight they may remain twice weekly until you are showing stable improvement. In Step Three, sessions will be held every two weeks.

Who does what?

Your therapist

As we said, you will never be told what to do—your therapist will merely act as your guide. They are there to educate you, encourage you, support you and keep you engaged and on track. They will have been highly trained in how best to help you and will have lots of useful tips and tricks that you can use to get well. They are not there to act as agents of your parents, and their only focus is for you to overcome your eating disorder. Talk to them if you have any problems or doubts, and they will do their best to help you get through them and come out the other side a happier and healthier person.

You

You should see treatment as *a chance for a fresh start*, a unique opportunity to break free from your eating disorder and begin a new, more satisfying life. Like any change, this may make you nervous, but you should concentrate on the potential benefits, including:

- Being able to think more freely, without being constantly oppressed by thoughts about eating, shape and weight
- Becoming a more cheerful, less irritable and rigid person
- Forming closer relationships with your loved ones and making new friends
- Being physically and mentally equipped to form your own family
- Expanding your sphere of interests and finding new things to enjoy
- Reclaiming your health and happiness

YOU NEED TO PLAY AN ACTIVE ROLE ACTIVE IN THE TREATMENT

You will be the one in the driving seat, so you will need to play an active role both during and between the sessions. It is you who will have to make the changes necessary to get well, and CBT-E treatment has little, if any, chance of success if you are not actively involved.

YOU SHOULD CONSIDER TREATMENT A PRIORITY

You are encouraged to shift your efforts from control of eating to succeeding at treatment. In other words, you should make your treatment a priority and put the same effort you devote to weight control into making positive changes.

GOOD TIMEKEEPING IS ESSENTIAL

It is of fundamental importance that each appointment starts and ends on time. Hence, it is a good idea to arrive a little early, about 10–15 minutes before each session. This will allow you to get comfortable, relax and mentally prepare things to discuss in the session.

IT IS CRUCIAL TO START WELL

The science tells us that the greater the changes you make in the early weeks, the more likely you are to be well one year down the line. Our patients who make a great effort to stop bingeing and purging straight away, for example, are usually free of this behaviour 12 months later. This is why you are encouraged to dive straight in, starting well and aiming to build what we call "therapeutic momentum." The idea is that once you've got over the initial hurdles, it should all be plainer sailing. In order to do this, of course, you will need to make the treatment a priority and work every day to make a change.

YOU SHOULD WORK TOGETHER WITH THE THERAPIST, JUST LIKE A TEAM

Your therapist cannot make you better without your input, and so you will need to let them know if anything is bothering you. Together you will discuss the features and maintenance mechanisms of your eating disorder, and they will ask you to do specific tasks between sessions (just like homework). Naturally, you will have to agree to do these tasks, but you should keep in mind that they are fundamental to your recovery and must be given absolute priority. It is precisely what you do between sessions that will determine how successful or not the treatment is.

YOU SHOULD AVOID INTERRUPTIONS IN TREATMENT

If you stop and start, or have breaks, you will not be able to build up therapeutic momentum—the head of steam you need to get over your eating disorder. No family holidays, no time off to study for exams. Before you start the programme, you should think ahead. Can you take these 20 weeks to get your life back? Once you decide to start treatment, it should become the most important thing in your life—nothing should stand in the way of your recovery.

Your parent(s), legal guardian(s) or significant other(s)

In our experience, your parents, or other people that you live with, can be a great help. They can support you through your CBT-E journey and help to create a home environment that will make it easier for you to make changes. For this reason, your therapist will discuss with you how best your parents or significant other could help you. If you are under the age of 18, they will be invited to attend a meeting lasting about 60 minutes on their own during the first week of treatment. The aim of this meeting will not be to discuss you behind your back, but instead to educate them on how to make your road to recovery easier. It is hard for parents to know what they should and shouldn't be doing, and so this meeting with your therapist will be of vital importance.

We find that giving them some pointers on how to behave at mealtimes, for example, will make them a lot less stressful experiences for you.

Later on, you may also want to enlist their help in implementing some of the treatment procedures, and your therapist may want to talk to you and your parents together for about 20 minutes immediately after some individual sessions with you. Remember that your therapist is acting for your benefit, not that of your parents, and the topics to be discussed with them will always be agreed upon by you beforehand.

CBT-E: the results

The effects of CBT-E on young patients have been assessed in scientific research conducted in the USA and by our team in Italy. These studies showed that two out of three patients who completed the treatment displayed a *significant increase in body weight* (when underweight at the start of treatment) and a *marked improvement in eating-disorder features*. These people were still in remission over a year later. If you dedicate yourself to the treatment, there is no reason why you should not recover from your eating disorder.

Here are some example stories of young people who have benefitted from the treatment. Like the other accounts in this book, these have been fictionalised but are based on the experiences of real patients.

Harry's story

My diagnosis was bulimia nervosa. It all started when I was 16. There were exams coming up at school, and I was worried I was going to fail. Academic achievement had always been important to my family, and I knew I was never going to measure up to my older brother's success. I started comfort eating while I revised, but eventually I was doing more bingeing than studying. I was also putting on weight, so I started eating less during meals. I cut down on bingeing a bit and started making myself sick afterwards. I was up and down like a yo-yo, and my exam prospects weren't getting any better, so my folks took me to a counsellor to help me deal with the stress in the lead-up to my exams. My body weight was stable, but low, and I was alternating full-on dieting with major bingeing. I was so ashamed and concerned about my weight that I was hiding away in my room all the time. I felt so bad that I started cutting myself to get some relief. It was clear that the sessions with my counsellor weren't doing any good, so I asked for something else. A friend of my father's is a psychiatrist, and he suggested CBT-E.

This was a life-saver. My therapist helped me to change my behaviour, one step at a time, starting with my bingeing and purging. Getting out of that cycle eventually made me feel a lot freer, and because I was not so ashamed of myself, I managed to leave my room and start hanging out with my mates again. Eating regularly made me feel like a normal person again and really increased my motivation. I wanted to change and take back control of my life, and through CBT-E I was able to do it. My grades suffered for a while there, but now I'm getting ready to do my leaving certificate and I'm feeling pretty confident. I might not get top marks, but I should do pretty well. I seldom think about my weight nowadays, and I feel much better about myself. I think the most useful bit of CBT-E for me was how it made me see that I was eating in response to stress and other negative emotions. I learned some really helpful, more productive strategies for coping with my emotions, and they no longer get the better of me. I am now a pro at identifying my triggers and dealing with them before they become a problem.

Leanne's story

I was diagnosed with anorexia nervosa when I was 14. I had already been in therapy with the rest of my family for about a year—we had been seeing a counsellor to sort out some relationship problems that we had been having. This didn't help me with my own problems though—when I was 13, I had gone on a strict diet because I had been teased about the shape of my butt by a classmate. It wasn't as if I was overweight, but I guess with all the trouble at home I was a bit sensitive to comments like that. Anyway, the upshot was that I lost a lot of weight, so much that my periods stopped. This was when my doctor suggested that I try CBT-E.

I was only eating fruit, vegetables and rice crackers by that time and basically never sat down. I would walk whenever I could, and it was really difficult for me to sit still and concentrate at school. I was absolutely terrified of getting fat and was constantly checking my body—looking in the mirror and squeezing my stomach and thighs—to make sure that I wasn't putting on any weight. My mood was all over the place. I was always thinking about food and snapping at my parents, which didn't help my family situation any. That was why it seemed a good idea to give CBT-E a shot, and I gradually began to put on weight and to spend less time thinking about food.

My fears went up a little during Step Two, when we started introducing avoided foods, but that soon passed. At the same time, we started working on my body image, and I managed to stop obsessively checking my appearance in the mirror and with my hands. Before I started monitoring, I hadn't realised just how much of that I was doing. Giving up self-monitoring during Step Three was a little scary, but my therapist helped me to understand that it wasn't something I could keep doing indefinitely, and so I would have to eventually give it up eventually. It made sense that I do that while I was still seeing him, so that if I had a meltdown, he'd be there to help me pick up the pieces. My periods had come back by that point, and my moods were much better. Although things were still a bit rocky at home, I was more able to deal with it, as I wasn't so irritable. I think it really helped that my mother got involved in my treatment. We were able to work on things together (with me in charge), which gave us something to focus on rather than just shouting at each other all the time.

I was still a bit sensitive, though, and towards the end of treatment I was worried that I wouldn't be able to handle comments about my weight, so we did a lot of work on that. We worked out strategies that I could use to prevent a relapse, and those really helped. Since then, I have managed to maintain a stable weight, and I enjoy myself a lot more. Because my therapist encouraged me to get out and try new things, I have a new group of friends, and they are really supportive. We are always doing something fun together, which gets me out of the house a lot. It also means that I always have something to look forward to, which is new for me. It's nice to be able to focus on my future plans without the chains of my eating disorder dragging me down.

FOR THE SCIENCE:

On the CBT-E website you will find an up-to-date list of the studies that have assessed the outcomes of CBT-E (www.cbte.co/research/efficacy-and-effectiveness/).

In summary

There is no magic wand solution to eating disorders. However, cognitive behavioural therapy is based on the belief that, given the right education and instructions, you can effectively cure yourself.

According to transdiagnostic cognitive behavioural theory, the key feature of all eating disorders is the overvaluation of shape, weight and eating (i.e., judging your self-worth mostly or only on your shape, weight and eating and/or your ability to control them). It is called the "core" feature, because it seems to reinforce and be reinforced by the other features (concerns about shape and weight, extreme weight-control behaviours, body checking and avoidance and feeling fat).

You may have one or more of four coexisting psychological and social problems that, according to our research, contribute to the maintenance of your eating disorder and interfere with treatment. These are: clinical perfectionism, core low self-esteem, marked interpersonal difficulties and mood intolerance. The broad form of CBT-E has extra modules to treat these problems alongside the eating disorder.

The main goal of CBT-E is to help you develop a healthier self-evaluation scheme—one not predominantly or exclusively based on shape, weight, eating and their control. To achieve this goal, the treatment adopts the following general strategies:

- Actively engaging you in the treatment and decision to change
- Gradually dismantling the psychological and behavioural features of your eating disorder
- Correcting the unhealthy mechanisms that maintain your eating disorder
- Making sure the changes are lasting

CBT-E requires that you play an active role during and between sessions to make the change. You must make your treatment a priority. It is crucial to start well and work together with your therapist, as a team, and avoid interruptions in treatment.

• Take-home message

CBT-E is a flexible, personalised treatment that can easily be adapted to suit your individual needs. However, if you sign up for CBT-E, you will be expected to play an active role in your own treatment—you will be the driver rather than the passenger. Your CBT-E treatment will be designed and driven by you. If you do the work, there is no reason why you it should not work for you. Take heart—there is light at the end of the tunnel, and you are already on your way to success!

Further reading

Dalle Grave, R., & Calugi, S. (2020). *Cognitive behavioural therapy for adolescents with eating disorders*. New York: Guilford Press.

Dalle Grave, R., Conti, M., Sartirana, M., Sermattei, S., & Calugi, S. (2021). Enhanced cognitive behaviour therapy for adolescents with eating disorders: A systematic review of current status and future perspectives. *IJEDO*, *3*, 1–11. doi:10.32044/ijedo.2021.01

Dalle Grave, R., & el Khazen, C. (2022). *Cognitive behaviour therapy for eating disorders in young people: A parents' guide*. London: Routledge.

Fairburn, C. G. (2008). *Cognitive-behavioral therapy of eating disorders*. New York: Guilford Press.

Fairburn, C. G. (2013). *Overcoming binge eating* (2nd ed.). New York: Guilford Press.

Fairburn, C. G., Cooper, Z., & Shafran, R. (2003). Cognitive behaviour therapy for eating disorders: A "transdiagnostic" theory and treatment. *Behaviour Research and Therapy*, *41*(5), 509–528. doi:10.1016/s0005-7967(02)00088-8

Part 2

Making the most of CBT-E

6

Getting ready

Before setting out on a long journey, it is a good idea to make a plan. Where will you be going? How will you get there? Where will you stay? If you organise your trip well, you will likely get where you need to when you need to—you minimise the risk of something going wrong. For the same reasons, it is important you prepare yourself before starting CBT-E. If you have read Part 1 of this book, you can already cross the number 1 off the preparation checklist that follows. If you haven't, or haven't for a while, you should definitely do that now.

Preparation checklist

1. Read Part 1 of the book.
2. Weigh up the pros and cons of starting Step One.
3. Decide whether you are ready to start.
4. Read the ten tips for getting the best out of CBT-E.

Weighing up the pros and cons of starting Step One

You are probably a bit uncertain about starting treatment, especially if you haven't been unwell for very long. There may be some things you would like to change, like binge-eating, but other habits, like strict dieting or exercising, you would like to keep. Alternatively, you may be highly motivated to start the programme but terrified of what you might lose or miss out on.

This is all okay. Remember that you won't be asked to make any changes immediately, so you can take a deep breath and relax. Step One of CBT-E is mainly dedicated to easing you into the programme. First, you and your therapist will work together to increase your understanding of the psychological mechanisms that are maintaining your eating disorder. Then, you will discuss together how the ways you are thinking and acting are affecting your life,

DOI: 10.4324/9781003342489-8

Table 6.1 Example list of pros and cons of starting Step One

My reasons NOT to start CBT-E	*My reasons TO start CBT-E*
I will have to work hard, and I'm afraid I won't make it.	*I'm tired of feeling miserable and cold all the time.*
A previous treatment failed (although it was very different as it was focused on weight regain without my agreement).	*I want my old life back.*
If I fail, I will disappoint my parents.	*I will improve my understanding of the psychological mechanisms maintaining my eating problem.*
I'm afraid of losing the sense of realisation I feel when I lose weight.	*I will learn how to interpret weight changes and perhaps reduce my concerns about my weight.*
	I will be in a better position to decide whether or not to address weight regain.
	I'll stop creating trouble for my parents.
	I like this programme because it doesn't ask me to do things I don't see as a problem, and helps me understand my eating disorder.

and whether you would like to change them. If your body weight is low, you will spend some time thinking about starvation symptoms and considering the implications of regaining some weight. If you experience frequent binge-eating episodes, you will begin to focus on improving your eating control. In both cases you will learn how to interpret your body weight correctly.

It will not be until the end of Step One that you will be asked to make the decision to change, but we are getting ahead of ourselves—what you need to focus on in the preparation phase are the advantages and disadvantages of starting Step One. Reasons for and against starting treatment are different for everyone, so take your time to think about it. Fill in a pros and cons table like the one shown as an example in Table 6.1. Do not complete this task at once, but go back to it a few times over the coming days. Reflect on each point and analyse your pros and cons critically and objectively. Consider the unique opportunity you will have in Step One to learn about the nature of your eating disorder. This will ultimately put you in a better position to understand the implications of change.

Deciding whether you are ready to start

To achieve the best results, you will need to prioritise this programme and put off anything that could interfere with it. If you are going on vacation or have other important commitments like exams coming up that you can't postpone, you would do better to start the programme later on. Remember that you will have two sessions a week in the first four weeks, and that there should be no interruptions throughout the programme. Therapeutic momentum is vital for success, and you need to maximise your chances, so if you cannot practically commit, perhaps now is not the right time for you.

As far as being mentally ready is concerned, by now you should have realised that you have nothing to lose by starting Step One, except for a couple of hours a week. Hours, however, that you will likely find very interesting and informative. All you need to do to be ready is be interested in what is happening to you and willing to talk about it. Go on! What are you waiting for? Cross the third item off the checklist!

Ten tips for making the best out of CBT-E

1. *Start well.* The data tells us that the size of the change achieved in the first four weeks of treatment is the most important predictor of the outcome one year after it's finished. For this reason, you are strongly encouraged to give it your all from the beginning. A positive attitude and a running start will get you the best results from the programme.
2. *Consider your treatment a priority.* Your treatment must be your number one priority. Indeed, it is probably the most important thing that you will ever do in your life. The more you engage, the better your chances of recovery.
3. *Play an active role.* You must play an active role in the treatment. In Step One this will involve you doing your best to understand how your eating disorder works, and in Step Two this will entail applying the strategies and procedures suggested by your therapist. The more effort you put in, the more you will get out of it.
4. *Consider the programme as a fresh start.* Look at the programme as a chance to start a new and healthy life. Wouldn't you like to become a new you, no longer burdened by your eating disorder?
5. *Dedicate the necessary time.* It takes time to change the way you think and behave. Think of the treatment as a marathon rather than a sprint.
6. *Follow the programme step by step.* Proceed at the suggested pace, don't rush—haste is the enemy of learning. Sometimes it is preferable to take a week or two to get something right. If you make a misstep or are having a trying time with a particular procedure, it might be best for you to take a step back to regroup. Slow and steady wins the race.
7. *Avoid interruptions.* There must be as few breaks as possible during the treatment, if any at all. This is especially important in the early weeks. Interrupting the treatment is destructive because it affects the therapeutic momentum and the opportunity to implement early change. Think of pushing a shopping cart up a hill. What would happen if you let it go halfway up?
8. *Be consistent.* To achieve remission from the eating disorder, it is essential to keep putting one foot in front of the other, day after day. You will

probably often feel frustrated and find it challenging to use the CBT-E procedures, especially when you first start. A general rule of thumb, though, is that the more difficult it seems to you to do something, the more important it is that you make the utmost effort to do it. This is the only way to interrupt the vicious cycles that are chaining you to your eating disorder.

9. *Don't expect easy and steady progress*. No matter how much effort you put in, there will be days when everything seems to go wrong. The trick is to take a deep breath and look at how much you have achieved so far. Everybody has a bad day, and temporary setbacks are to be expected. Your therapist will be able to teach you how to get over these bumps in the road. The important thing to ask yourself is whether you are making progress overall. If you are, it is only logical to continue.
10. *Adopt the following motto*. "It might be hard, but it'll be worth it."

In summary

Step One will give you a unique opportunity to understand the nature of your eating disorder and put you in a better position to weigh up the implications of change. It's good to be prepared, however, so before starting the programme, you should:

1. Read Part 1 of the book.
2. Weigh up the pros and cons of starting Step One.
3. Decide whether you are ready to start.
4. Read the ten tips for getting the best out of CBT-E.

• Take-home message

Only you can decide when you are ready to learn about your eating disorder, but rest assured, you really do have nothing to lose—no one will make you do anything you do not agree to.

7

Overview of the three steps

Step One—starting well and deciding to change

Once you decide to sign up to the programme, you will be able to start. Step One of CBT-E has a duration of three to four weeks, two sessions per week, and the following aims:

- Increasing your understanding of your eating disorder
- Reducing your weight concerns
- Reducing your binge-eating episodes (if applicable)
- Deciding to make a change

If you are low weight, this Step also includes choosing to tackle weight regain (which you will do in Step Two).

To achieve these objectives, the following procedures are implemented:

- Creating your personal formulation
- Establishing real-time self-monitoring
- Collaborative weekly weighing
- Using the Eating Problem Check List (EPCL)
- Establishing regular eating
- Thinking about change
- Getting your parents on board

As a general rule, you will work on the procedures in the order shown in Table 7.1.

The EPCL and the other procedures will be described in detail in the following chapters.

The sessions

Each CBT-E session last about 50 minutes, except for the first, which may last as long as 90 minutes, so the procedures can be explained. How this

DOI: 10.4324/9781003342489-9

Table 7.1 Suggested content of Step One sessions

Weeks:	*1*	*2*	*3*	*4*
Personal formulation	√			
Real-time self-monitoring	√	√	√	√
Collaborative weekly weighing	√	√	√	√
Eating Problem Check List (EPCL)		√	√	√
Establishing regular eating		√	√	√
Thinking about change			√	√
Involving parents	√*	√**	√**	

Notes: * Parent-only session (if you are under the age of 18)
* Joint sessions with you and your parents

time is divided between tasks will vary on a case-by-case basis, as how much input is required to thoroughly review the treatment procedures will vary from patient to patient. That being said, the approximate time frames (in brackets) devoted to the various tasks in the CBT-E sessions are the following:

1. In-session weighing and filling in the Eating Problem Check List (5 minutes)
2. Reviewing your monitoring records and homework (about 10–15 minutes)
3. Setting the agenda for the session (a few minutes)
4. Working through the items in the agenda (25 minutes)
5. Summarising the session, agreeing on homework and arranging the next appointment (5 minutes)

Review sessions—taking stock

"Taking Stock" is introduced in a review session after the end of Step One if you are not low weight, and at flexible intervals (usually every four weeks) during Step Two if you are addressing weight regain. These sessions will be partially dedicated to reviewing your progress, identifying any problems you are having, modifying your formulation as needed and planning the next four weeks. Besides these tasks, each review session has two main purposes:

1. To identify the obstacles to change if you having any difficulties. This is important because unless we get to the bottom of the problem, you are unlikely to get a good result.
2. To understand how your eating disorder may have changed. Your treatment can then be adapted in line with your progress and/or difficulties.

Step Two—making the change

In Step Two, you will continue the procedures you started in Step One—self-monitoring, weekly weighing and regular eating—and also learn new ones designed to help you:

1. Address the psychological and behavioural features of your eating disorder
2. Address the factors that are maintaining your eating disorder
3. Develop the skills to cope with setbacks

How Step Two unfolds will be determined by the features of your eating disorder. For example, if you are not low weight, Step Two will involve 8–9 weekly sessions, while if you are low weight, the sessions will continue twice a week until your weight regain trend is consistent. After that, the frequency of Step Two sessions will be once a week. Hence, the number of sessions in Step Two will depend on how low your body weight is and the difficulties you encounter in regaining weight.

Step Two includes one or more of the following modules, which are used to address the processes that maintain your eating disorder:

- Low weight and undereating
- Excessive exercising
- Purging
- Body image
- Dietary rules
- Events, moods and eating
- Setbacks and mindsets

Step Two is highly flexible and adaptable, and the procedures involved will depend on the features of your eating disorder and the changes that occur during the treatment.

Step Three—ending well

Step Three is the final stage in treatment and is concerned with ending the treatment well. Ending well is just as important as starting well, as Step Three is designed to prepare you for life after the programme. As such, it has two main goals:

1. To ensure that the changes made in treatment are maintained afterwards
2. To minimise the risk of relapse

In addition, any concerns you may have about ending treatment will need to be addressed, and certain treatment procedures phased out.

Step Three consists of three appointments held two weeks apart. The usual session structure is retained throughout, but the sessions become progressively more future-oriented and less concerned with the present.

In most cases, treatment can, and should, end on time. There are circumstances under which it is appropriate to offer more treatment or extend it, but in our experience, these are not common. As long as you have got to the point where you have managed to disrupt your main maintenance mechanisms, and the house of cards that is your eating disorder is beginning to collapse, you will continue to improve after treatment has ended. Under these circumstances, treatment can be wound up, and it is in your interest that it is. Otherwise, you might think that the further improvements you make are due to the ongoing therapy rather than your own empowered self.

Step Three has four components:

1. Addressing concerns about ending treatment
2. Ensuring that progress is maintained
3. Phasing out certain treatment procedures
4. Minimising the risk of relapse in the long term

The strategies and procedures involved are described in detail in Chapter 23.

Post-treatment review sessions

At the end of your CBT-E programme, you won't just be pushed out the door, into the cold—post-treatment review sessions will be scheduled 4, 12 and 20 weeks after the end of treatment. The purpose of these is to see how you are doing and whether there is anything we can do to help. During these sessions, you and your therapist will review your progress, revise your long-term maintenance plan and, if necessary (e.g., if you have not resumed regular periods), weigh up the pros and cons of further weight gain.

In summary

CBT-E for young people is organised in three steps and includes review sessions during and after the treatment.

Step One

Step One lasts three to four weeks, has two sessions per week, and will help you understand your eating disorder, reduce your weight concerns and any binge-eating and decide to make a change (including weight regain).

Step Two

The content and duration of Step Two will depend on your eating disorder presentation. It includes the following modules as applicable:

- Low weight and undereating
- Excessive exercising
- Purging
- Body image
- Dietary rules
- Events, moods and eating
- Setbacks and mindsets

Step Three

Step Three consists of three appointments held two weeks apart and has the aims of ensuring that the changes you have made last and minimising the risk of relapse.

Review sessions

They are held after the end of Step One if you are not low weight, and at flexible intervals (usually every four weeks) during Step Two if you are low weight.

Post-treatment review sessions

They are held 4, 12 and 20 weeks after the end of the programme.

• Take-home message

The length and content of you personalised CBT-E programme will depend on your individual needs and progress. However, it is not designed to go on indefinitely. Once you have learned and practised the skills you need to overcome your eating disorder, you will be free to enjoy your wonderful new life!

8

Creating your personal formulation

As we saw in Chapter 5, your personal formulation is a visual representation of the mechanisms maintaining your eating disorder in the form of a flow chart. This is one of the first tasks that you will work on with your therapist during your first CBT-E session. You will concentrate on only the main, most powerful mechanisms that seem to be maintaining your eating disorder—you don't want to get bogged down in the details. Your first formulation is provisional and will be updated periodically throughout the programme, as you and your therapists learn more about your maintenance mechanisms. You can practice building your personal formulation by yourself by following the steps described next.

The first step is to *identify your eating disorder's main psychological and behavioural features* by answering the questions in Table 8.1 Think about which of these have been true for you over the past four weeks.

The second step is to draw up your own personal formulation. Look at the examples in Figure 8.1. One is drawn by Alex, who is not underweight but experiences binge-eating episodes and compensatory self-induced vomiting, and one by Bethany, who is low weight and is experiencing several starvation symptoms.

Now write down the features of your eating disorder you have identified in the boxes of Figure 8.2. This already has placeholder mechanisms in light grey. All you need to do is go over the ones that apply to you and the relevant arrows in a darker colour, ignoring the ones that don't. Before you do this, if you are low weight you should brush up on the starvation symptoms we discussed in Chapter 3. Pay special attention to the section on the Minnesota Starvation Experiment and the symptoms of being low weight and undereating (listed in Table 3.1). Write in the low weight box the symptoms you are experiencing due to being underweight that you did not have before you lost the weight. During treatment you will draw this on a separate sheet of paper and put it in an empty ring binder.

DOI: 10.4324/9781003342489-10

Table 8.1 How many of these eating disorder features have applied to you in the last four weeks?

Features of my eating disorder	*Yes*	*No*
Overvaluation of shape and weight *How I see myself depends mainly or only on my shape and weight.*		
Overvaluation of eating control *How I see myself depends mainly or only on my ability to control my eating.*		
Dietary restriction *I follow a strict diet, skip meals and/or avoid certain foods.*		
Binge eating *I sometimes find myself eating a lot more than I intended to without being able to stop.*		
Self-induced vomiting *I sometimes make myself sick after meals.*		
Laxative misuse *I use laxatives to control my weight.*		
Diuretic misuse *I use water pills to control my weight.*		
Excessive exercising *I exercise to control my weight, shape or amount of fat, or to burn extra calories.*		
Low weight *My BMI is below 19 or the corresponding for-age centile.*		
Events and moods influencing eating *I sometimes find myself eating when something bad happens or I feel bad.*		

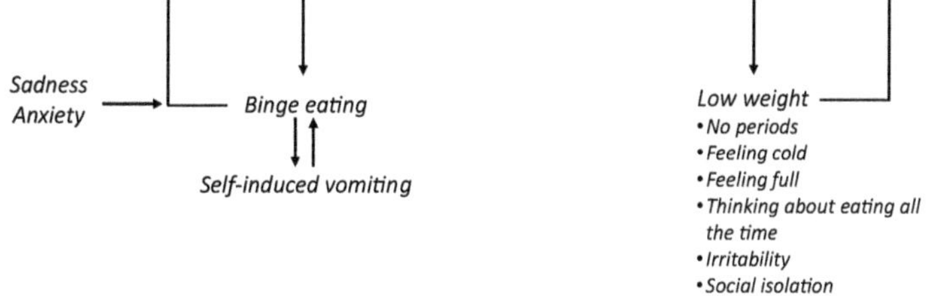

Figure 8.1 Example of personal formulations drawn by a not-underweight person (Alex) and an underweight person (Bethany)

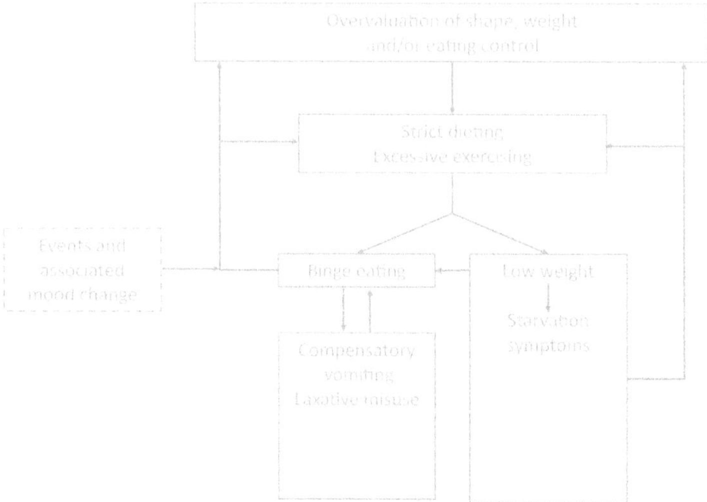

Figure 8.2 Use this diagram to build your own personal formulation

The third step is to go back to Chapter 3 to study how the features of your eating disorder that you have identified and included in your personal formulation are maintaining your eating disorder. For example, if you have a strict diet, you should read about how this reinforces your eating-disorder mindset.

The final step is to analyse the implications of your personal formulation. The most critical point to think about is that in the process of getting well, you will address not only the things you want to get rid of, for example binge-eating episodes and starvation symptoms, but also the mechanisms that are responsible for maintaining them, such as strict dieting, low weight, events and moods influencing eating and overvaluation of shape, weight and eating control. Hopefully, your formulation will help you to visualise the vicious cycles that are operating in your eating disorder and the chains that will need to be broken if you are to be free.

Sara's story

I was 16 years old and in high school when I first went on a diet. I didn't like the way I looked in my bikini so I decided to lose a bit of weight to get ready for the summer. I didn't go overboard, and lost 4 kg in about two months. I was happy with the results and managed to stay that way for several months. However, when the first COVID-19 pandemic lockdown hit, I kind of went off the rails. I was stuck at home with my parents and older brother, and my sister was away at university in another city. I didn't know what to do with myself, and I would find myself pacing around my room all day. I began to fixate on my food intake and exercise regime, which kind of gave a structure to my day. At first, I felt better, more in control of what was going on, but soon the weight began to fall off me, and in a few months' time, it had dropped to 40 kg. My parents freaked out and took me to a local clinic, where they put me in treatment. To be honest, I just kind of switched off. I didn't really understand what was going on, and I felt like everyone was treating me like a child again—"do this, don't do that . . ." They said that my eating disorder was like a disease that could be cured if I did what they told me to, but I didn't get any better.

This is why my parents set up a consultation at a CBT-E clinic. At the beginning, I only went to please them. I didn't really believe that they could help me. My earlier treatment had done nothing for me at all, and I didn't see the point of starting all over again. The therapist was nice though, so I said I'd tell her about my problem, although at that time I didn't really see it as a problem at all. The fact that I had managed to lose the weight I set out to made me feel confident. I felt that my relationships and my life in general had actually improved since I lost the weight. So, I had no doubt at all in saying that eating control and low weight was a choice when my therapist asked me if I thought it was a choice or a problem. However, talking to my therapist did kind of make me think, especially when she asked me whether I would be able to relax my eating and exercising for a few days. She said that she didn't consider the eating disorder like a disease, but instead as a consequence of the way I thought about myself. She said that people with eating disorders tend not to see their behaviour as a problem, because the disorder itself makes you feel that way—like a fish in a tank, who has forgotten what the ocean is like. She showed me how my low weight was actually leading me down a path to ill health, feeding into my eating disorder. Together we drew up something called a provisional formulation, which showed the ways that my dietary restriction and exercising were making it difficult for me to focus on anything but my weight and eating. This made sense to me, as I remember when I was preparing for a violin exam, and all I could think about at that time was that. My grades even started to slip for a while there until it was over.

The therapist then asked me what my reasons for not doing treatment were. This was good, because she actually wanted to hear my opinion, but once I had listed my reasons for and against treatment in writing, I had to admit to myself that the benefits of not starting therapy were a little silly. Another good thing was that she explained to me exactly what CBT-E involved, and that I would be in control—not her or my parents.

Also, she said that I wouldn't have to do anything to change my weight straight away, which was kind of a big relief. I learned a lot during that session and agreed to go to the next one in a week's time, after I had thought about what we discussed. During that time, I realised that I had nothing to lose, so I decided to start CBT-E Step One.

In summary

Your personal formulation is a visual representation of your main eating-disorder features (boxes) and maintenance mechanisms (arrows). The formulation maps the way these features interact, and therefore the mechanisms that maintain the eating disorder and need to be disrupted by treatment. You will build it collaboratively with your therapist during your first CBT-E session, and it will be updated periodically as your eating disorder evolves.

• Take-home message

Your personal formulation is a road map that will guide your treatment towards recovery from your eating disorder.

9

Real-time self-monitoring

The monitoring record is introduced in the first CBT-E session and considered the most important tool of the programme. Filling it in properly is as important as attending the sessions.

The monitoring record may be used to help you monitor:

- Your weight change
- Eating behaviour
- Excessive exercising
- Binge-eating episodes
- Purging behaviours
- Body checking and/or avoidance
- Other behaviours caused by your eating behaviour
- Influential events, thoughts and emotions

To work, your monitoring record must be filled out in "real time" that is, at the precise moment in which you enact a behaviour, or you feel a thought or an emotion. It is different from a food diary in this respect, because a food diary is normally filled in at the end of each meal or in the evening, not in real time. Moreover, the monitoring record is used to record not only the food you eat but also the events, thoughts and emotions you experience.

The purpose of real-time self-monitoring is twofold:

1. *It provides a detailed picture of how you behave*, helping you get an accurate picture of how your eating disorder operates. This is because reporting relevant behaviours, thoughts, emotions and events as they happen minimises errors that would otherwise occur if you had to rely on your memory at the end of the meal or in the evening. In addition, it gives you and the therapist a great opportunity to check the maintenance processes on your formulation. Armed with the information from your monitoring record, you can confirm the first version or update it with new information.

DOI: 10.4324/9781003342489-11

2. *It makes you more aware of what you are doing at the precise moment you do it.* This makes it easier for you to notice, and ultimately put a stop to, behaviours that initially seem automatic and out of control. Noticing a behaviour as it happens gives you a valuable opportunity to decide not to do it, and if you record the events, thoughts or emotions that preceded that behaviour, it gives you real insight into potential triggers.

Doing real-time monitoring accurately and honestly is fundamental to the programme's success. At first, writing down everything you eat and think can be annoying, but after a few days, it will become second nature. We have yet to encounter anyone whose lifestyle made it truly impossible to monitor. Regard it as a challenge. When you talk over what you have written with your therapist, you will see just how helpful it can be.

How to use the monitoring record

Look at the example monitoring record filled in by Emma to see how to monitor (Figure 9.1). A new record (or records) should be started each day.

In **column 1**, you will write down the *time* you eat or drink anything.

EMMA'S MONITORING RECORD

Day Friday **Date** April 23rd

Time	Food and drinks consumed	Place	*	V/L/E	Context and comments
5:30	1 glass of water	Kitchen			I woke up early.
12:39	1 bowl of salad 1 apple }	Kitchen			I am in control.
3:30					I argued with mom; she does not understand me. I feel fat and irritated.
4:00	3 ice-creams 2 packets of chips 5 chocolate-chip cookies	Bedroom	* * *		
				V	I have no willpower. I'm disgusted with myself.
8:00	1 cup of salad 1 apple 4 glasses of water }	Kitchen			Mom told me off because I didn't eat the meat. She doesn't understand me. I am angry, and I feel fat. Dad encourages me to eat at normal speed, but all he really wants is for me to eat more.

Figure 9.1 An example of a daily monitoring record filled in by Emma

Note: V = vomiting; L = laxative misuse; E = exercise

In **column 2**, you will write down *what you eat and drink*. Don't count calories, just make a simple (non-technical) note of the food and drink you consume. Each item should be written in the monitoring record immediately after swallowing them, not at the end of the meal. This is why you should keep your monitoring record on the table where you eat. You should always carry that day's monitoring record with you, so that you can record anything you eat or drink between meals in real time. Remembering what you ate and drank a few hours later is not good enough because it cannot help you change your behaviour. Meals should be identified using brackets, any other food or drink without.

In **column 3**, you will list *where* you consumed the food or drink. If you ate or drank at home, specify the room.

In **column 4**, you should put an asterisk (*) next to every food or drink that you felt was too much. This should be your opinion. What anyone else might think is not important. It is essential that you record all food you eat during binges and identify them with asterisks in this column.

In **column 5**, you should record when you vomit (write "V"), take laxatives (write "L" and the number of pills taken) or exercise (write "E"). Specify how long you exercised and what you did in column 6.

Column 6 should be used to record the events, thoughts and emotions that you feel have affected your behaviour. For example, if an event triggered an episode of binge eating, you should report it in this column. Here you can also write down important events that did not affect your eating. It's a good idea to note all the intense emotions you feel when you feel them, whether they influenced your eating or not. Write "sad" if you feel sadness, "anxious" if you feel anxiety and so on for boredom, loneliness, feeling fat or concerns about eating, weight or body shape. Column 6 should also be used to record your weight each time you measure it.

With practice, real-time self-monitoring will help you record when your eating-disorder mindset is triggered and how it makes you act in the very moment that this happens.

There is a blank monitoring record (Table 28.1) in the CBT-E TOOLS at the back of this book. Your therapist will give you several copies of this, but if you want, you can make photocopies of it directly, or download it using the QR code:

You could even make your own version on the computer if you prefer. Don't draw one in a notepad—you have to use a new one every day. You should put all the monitoring records you have filled in in your ring binder. Keep them organised in date order so you can review your progress when you need to. Every treatment session will include a detailed review of your latest monitoring sheets. You must therefore remember to bring them with you!

FAQs and doubts about real-time self-monitoring—your questions answered

Can I use an app to monitor my eating?

We realise that you are used to using smartphone apps for a variety of purposes. However, you should use your paper CBT-E monitoring records and not an app, because we know they work well. Moreover, using a sheet of paper gives you enough space for detailed recording of your behaviours, thoughts and feelings and whatever else you need. Apps and notebooks, on the other hand, tend to restrict the quantity and type of the information that you can record, making them unfit for purpose.

Can I show my parents my monitoring records?

We suggest you don't let your parents see your monitoring records, as this might influence what you write down. Your monitoring record should be kept private, for discussion only with your therapist.

Do I really have to fill in my monitoring records during meals?

Yes. In addition to providing a more accurate record, real-time self-monitoring helps in two other ways. First, it helps you "step outside the moment," looking from an objective, de-centred perspective on your mealtime thoughts and feelings. This can help you understand what you are thinking and feeling, and at the same time makes your thoughts and feelings less intense. Second, by helping you notice what you are doing when you are doing it, real-time self-monitoring can help you interrupt some forms of automatic behaviour (e.g., eating too slowly or too fast, hiding food).

I'd be too embarrassed or ashamed to write down some of my feelings or behaviours

Don't worry! Your therapist will never judge your behaviours or feelings. Their job is to help you find effective strategies for tackling them. Honesty is the best policy.

It will make me even more preoccupied with eating than I am already

This may be true at first—writing down what you eat can increase your preoccupation with eating. However, these are constructive, not destructive, concerns because they will help you and your therapist to become more aware of your problematic eating behaviours and the processes that are maintaining them. Self-monitoring is a necessary step to you becoming an expert on your eating disorder. You will find that your concerns about eating usually vanish after a week or two.

Luisa's story

Looking back, I think the CBT-E procedure that most helped me was real-time self-monitoring. By the time I was referred for what I think of as proper treatment, my eating was all over the place. I had begun to pay more attention to my diet when I was 16 and I started high school. There were all these thin and pretty girls there, and I wanted to lose weight so that I could be like them. I didn't think that my new classmates would accept me the way I was. I started to cut things out of my diet and to exercise daily, and it was not long before I was eating only vegetables and my body weight had dropped dramatically. I ended up in hospital twice because of my weight loss and malnutrition, and once I got out, I had to go and see a psychiatrist and a nutritionist. They gave me antidepressants and antipsychotics and a special diet. I just felt numb and hungry all the time, so I ended up binge-eating and my weight went up.

Thankfully at that point I got referred for CBT-E. My therapist and I filled in a questionnaire about my eating habits and thoughts and feelings over the last month, and he told me that I was showing signs of overvaluation of shape and weight—which means that my shape and weight were more important to me than they should be. He explained that this was why I was so worried about my diet and suggested that I monitor what I was eating while I was doing it. This seemed like a bad idea to me at the time, because I wanted to stop thinking about food all the time, not to focus on it. My therapist explained to me, though, that while my eating concerns might get worse at first, if I stuck at it, they would pass, and I would begin to see the benefits of real-time self-monitoring, so I agreed to give it a try. He wasn't wrong, although it took me some time to see it! I remember when I first sat down to a meal with my monitoring records by my plate—it made me so anxious! I thought my therapist would be angry with me at my next session because I had given up self-monitoring before I'd even started, but he said, "Well done for trying!" and suggested we talk about why it had been difficult for me. I told him that I'd eaten far too much, and I would have been too ashamed to write down what I had actually eaten, so I stopped halfway through and tore up the paper. This made me feel so bad that I ate the rest of the pie that my mother had put in the fridge. My therapist said that this was important information to know, and that if I had another go at self-monitoring, we might learn even more about how my eating disorder mindset made me think and behave. The fact that he didn't judge me for my bingeing made me feel that he really was on my side, so I agreed to try again. This time I was much more successful, and eventually I began to see how real-time self-monitoring could help me to understand my binge-eating triggers. Seeing them written down in black and white made it clear to me that I would binge when I felt bad, like when I had an argument with my parents or didn't stick to my diet. Recognising these triggers in real time was the first gigantic step to getting over them, and in the end self-monitoring wasn't so difficult to do.

In summary

Real-time self-monitoring is a key procedure of CBT-E. It consists of recording relevant behaviours, thoughts, emotions and events in the moment that they are experienced on a specific monitoring record. It is not a food diary.

There are three main reasons why real-time self-monitoring procedure is employed in CBT-E:

1. It distances you from your immediate behaviour and helps you see that change is possible.
2. It highlights key behaviours, thoughts and feelings and the context in which they occur—you can see yourself enacting your formulation in real time.
3. It opens new avenues for change.

It is essential that you carry your monitoring record with you at all times so that you can write down the behaviour you are monitoring in real time. This minimises problems with recall and enables you to make changes there and then.

• Take-home message

Your monitoring record is a powerful weapon against your eating disorder. Use it wisely and use it well.

10

Collaborative weighing

Like many young people with an eating disorder, you probably have your own ideas about weight, particularly what is a healthy weight, and the causes of weight changes. However, what you believe may not reflect the facts. It is also likely that you are very concerned about your weight and the effects that the treatment will have on it. These preoccupations may prompt you to weigh yourself several times a day, or refuse to weigh yourself altogether. However, as we have seen, both weight checking and weight avoidance act to increase your weight concern and therefore maintain your eating disorder.

The facts about weight and weighing

Body weight **fluctuates** naturally day by day and over the course of the day or month (in girls with a regular cycle) because of changes in hydration status. In fact, about 60% of our body weight is made up of water. Just like the ocean tides, your body weight will rise and then fall.

> JARGON BUSTER
>
> **fluctuate** (verb): go up and down

Body fat, on the other hand, makes up a much smaller percentage of our bodies and takes much longer to deposit and burn off. Therefore, if you weigh yourself several times a day, all you are actually doing is working yourself up over temporary changes in water content. If your water weight goes down, you may feel triumphant, but your "victory" is, in fact, a hollow one. If your water weight goes up, this too is meaningless, but is likely trigger feelings of disappointment or despair. It may fuel your eating disorder by prompting you to step up your efforts to cut back on calories, or lead to a binge-eating episode through all-or-nothing thinking: "What's the point. All my efforts have been for nothing because I have put on weight. I might as well give up and eat what I want."

As you already know by now, the binge may provide temporary relief from the sense of failure provoked by a water weight gain but will then itself cause

DOI: 10.4324/9781003342489-12

a crushing sense of defeat. All weight checking does is fuel the cycle, making your eating disorder worse.

At the other end of the spectrum, avoiding weighing prevents you from getting accurate information on how your weight is changing. This may cause your imagination to run wild and your weight loss or gain to get out of hand. Weight avoidance maintains your fear of weight and puts up a barrier to changing your eating habits.

But how do I stop myself?

We help you reduce your weight concerns through a procedure we call collaborative weighing. Collaborative weighing is a cornerstone of the CBT-E programme and is introduced in the second session of CBT-E.

The first thing you will do is weigh yourself in the therapist's office. They will help you to calculate your BMI. However, since it is an easy task, you can do it by yourself as follows:

My weight (kg) _____: my height (m^2) ______= ______ my BMI

If you know your weight in pounds and your height in inches, the ratio in this equation must be multiplied by 703.

Fast Fact

The threshold for considering adults as having significantly low weight is debated and varies, but a BMI of below 18.5 is the most frequently used. However, in teens, BMI is age- and sex-specific, and is often referred to as BMI-for-age percentile (see www.cdc.gov/healthyweight/assessing/bmi/childrens_bmi/about_childrens_bmi.html). In people with an eating disorder, we recommend considering a BMI of 19.0, or the corresponding BMI-for-age percentile in those who are under 16 (your therapist will help you to identify this), as the minimum threshold for a healthy weight, because below this BMI most people experience some adverse physical and psychosocial effects of being underweight (starvation symptoms).

You will write your weight on your monitoring record. Then, your therapist will explain to you what your weight means and talk to you about the information in the following sections. Collaborative weighing involves weighing yourself weekly, with your therapist, and talking together about the number on the scales. You will ultimately become an expert in interpreting changes in your own weight. Other than that, the procedure has five main goals:

1. To correct your misconceptions about weight changes
2. To provide reliable information about your weight
3. To help you to interpret the number on the scales correctly
4. To address frequent weight checking and/or weight avoidance
5. To reduce your weight concerns

Information about weight change

Wanting to have an exact weight all the time is like wanting to have a constant heart rate. As we said, the number on the scale fluctuates during the day due to modifications in the body's water content, which accounts for about 60% of total body weight. The main cause of short-term weight variations is changes in hydration status. This is why boxers may stop eating and drinking before a fight if they are trying to "make weight." They aren't actually losing body weight, just water weight.

As water weight fluctuates naturally, it is almost impossible to maintain a constant body weight. So, when you set your weight goals, you should bear this in mind. It is pointless fixating on a particular number on the scales. Instead, you should factor in a range of about 3 kilograms (6 pounds). This will allow for natural weight fluctuations that have nothing to do with changes in energy supply. Do not fall into the trap of thinking that changes in your weight are changes in your body fat—they are mainly due to variations in hydration status.

Single scale readings can be deceptive and not indicative of changes in weight. To correctly interpret weight change, you should learn to look at the trend in your weight over 3–4 weeks by referring to your weight chart (see below) rather than concentrating on the latest single reading. Indeed, a single reading is almost impossible to interpret because of its uncertainty. For this reason, therapists will always remind you that it is impossible to interpret a single reading. As shown in Figure 10.1, to correctly interpret your weight trend you need to look at least 3–4 weekly readings.

Once-a-week collaborative weighing

There are two main things that your therapist will teach you about weighing:

1. How to interpret the number on the scales
2. The adverse effects of weighing avoidance and frequent weight checking

To this end, you will weigh yourself collaboratively (with your therapist) once a week at the beginning of the session. In most cases, you will start the procedure in the second session and continue until Step Three of the treatment, when you will start to weigh yourself alone at home.

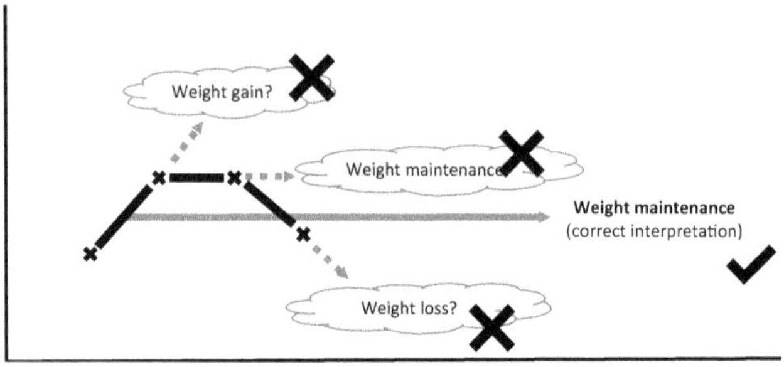

Figure 10.1 How to interpret changes in your weight on your weight chart

The collaborative weighing procedure involves the following three components:

1. *Weighing and recording*. Once a week, at the beginning of each session, you will measure your weight with your therapist. You should say the number on the scales out loud and let your therapist check it so that you agree. Then, you and the therapist will plot the reading on your weight chart (see below).
2. *Interpretation*. A single reading is meaningless, and so each week you and your therapist will jointly interpret the emerging trend by examining the last four weeks' readings. Is the line going up, down or remaining stable?
3. *Consistency*. This procedure should be repeated week by week. Regular, collaborative weighing and accurate interpretation will reduce your weight concerns and may help you change your eating habits.

You should not weigh yourself outside of sessions until Step Three of the treatment, when you start weighing yourself at home. If you have scales at home and you have difficulties resisting the urge to jump on, we suggest that you use a "coping card" to remind you of your reasons for not weighing yourself (see Chapter 22). If you do give in to the urge, you should record this on your monitoring record, together with the events, thoughts and emotions that led you to check your weight. Please note that we advise you and your parents not to hide the scales, because you must learn to manage the urge to weigh yourself.

Fast Fact

The scales used by CBT-E therapists has intervals of 0.5 kg (or 1 pound). We recommend avoiding electronic or overly precise scales (e.g., measuring 100–200 g intervals) as they will be more likely to trigger unhelpful worries about tiny changes in water weight.

Your weight chart

The individualised weight chart is prepared by your therapist and includes the number of weeks on the horizontal axis and the number of weight in kilograms (or pounds) on the vertical axis. Your initial weight value will usually be approximately halfway up the vertical axis if you are not low weight. In contrast, the value will be along the lower part of the axis if you are low weight. Your therapist will also draw a dashed line representing your minimum healthy weight threshold. This will be equivalent to your BMI of 19, or the corresponding BMI-for-age percentile if you are under 16.

Each week with your therapist, you will mark your weight reading in the row for the corresponding week. Then, your therapist will ask you to interpret your weight trend over the last four weeks rather than concentrating on the latest single reading. It might be helpful also you try to adopt the mindset of a person who does not have an eating disorder by asking yourself: "If I were a person who does not have an eating disorder, how would I interpret my weight?" You should also write the weight number and interpretation in column 6 of your monitoring record (e.g., "48 kg, my weight is stable").

Figure 10.2 shows an example of a weight chart belonging Maria, an underweight girl, filled in in Step One of the CBT-E. As you can see, the therapist has drawn a dashed line corresponding to her BMI of 19.0, which is the minimum weight she should be to be healthy, and the four measurements of her weight in Step One.

There is a blank weight chart (Table 28.3) in the CBT-E TOOLS at the back of this book. Your therapist will provide you with one of your own, but if you want to practice you can photocopy the one in this book or download it using the QR code:

Effects of treatment on weight

You are probably feeling anxious about how the treatment will affect your weight. However, *if you are not low weight* (i.e., you have a BMI equal to or greater than 19.0 or the corresponding BMI-for-age percentile if you are under 16), you will probably not experience significant weight changes. Some people do gain a little weight, but it is not possible to predict precisely what will happen to you. Our body weight is determined partly by our genes, and it therefore is very challenging to modify it.

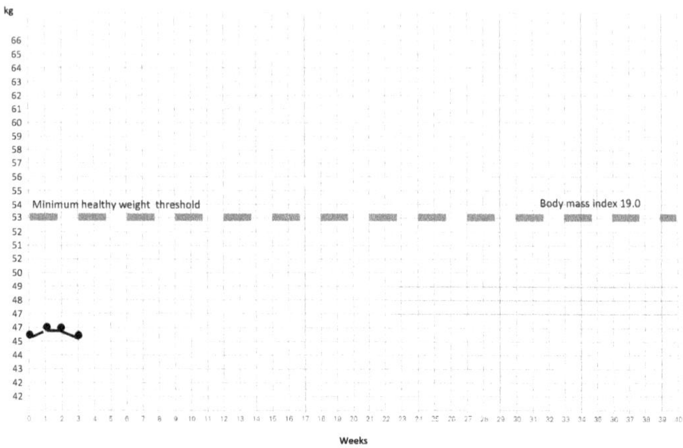

Figure 10.2 The weight chart filled in by Maria, an underweight 17-year-old, during Step One of CBT-E

However, remember that one of the main aims of CBT-E is to give you control over your eating, which will in turn give you as much control over your weight as possible. For this reason, we suggest you postpone the decision on what weight range to aim for until near the end of the programme. At this point, both your eating habits and your weight should be stable, and you should be able to follow flexible healthy eating guidelines without adopting extreme weight-control behaviours. As we have seen, dietary restraint reinforces preoccupation with food and eating, making binge-eating more likely. This is why we suggest letting go of your weight loss goals for now. You need to be able to weigh yourself dispassionately, scientifically, without being invested in the number on the scales.

If you are low weight (i.e., you have a BMI under 19 or the corresponding BMI-for-age percentile if you are under 16), once you have decided to make the change and attempt weight regain, the goal of the treatment is for you to gradually reach and maintain a weight range of 3 kilograms (6 pounds) over your BMI of 19. Your "new normal" weight should fulfil the following four conditions (see also the Low Weight and Undereating module):

1. It can be maintained without adopting extreme weight-control behaviours.
2. It does not cause starvation symptoms (see Chapter 3).
3. It is compatible with physical health and normal development.
4. It lets you have a social life.

Remember too that if you are a teen or young adult, you have likely not stopped growing yet, even if your physical development has stopped or slowed due to undereating and low weight. This means that your weight restoration may allow you to start growing again, and the weight goals you used to have will no longer be applicable.

Marcus's story

When I was 15, I met a guy I liked, but he didn't even know I existed. I thought he'd like me better if I got in shape, so I had my mom send me to a nutritionist. I stuck to the diet she gave me for a couple of months, but then I thought I could speed things up if I cut down even more on the carbs and went more often to the gym. My weight got so low and I was so obsessed with it that that my mom made me see a CBT-E therapist. I managed to start eating at regular times like the therapist suggested, but when he wanted to me to stop weighing myself at home I panicked. By that time, I was weighing myself once a day and planning my eating and exercising around the number on the scales (which was 56 kg, by the way)—I'd be like, "No carbs and more walking for you!" if it hadn't gone down. I got that my weight had basically taken over my life and that weighing myself every day was making it worse, but it was so hard to stop! The first week I was only able to not weigh myself on one day, and that day my anxiety was over the top! I told this to my therapist, and we talked about water weight and the fact that actual body weight cannot change on a daily basis. He told me that by weighing myself every day at home I was making it more difficult for me to stick to my planned meals and snacks, that I was making sure that I would worry about my weight every day. He suggested that I concentrate on sticking to my regular eating plan, and that it would be better to wait to weigh myself once a week in my therapist's office, where we could talk together about the actual meaning of the number on the scales. That actually helped me a whole lot! Over time, not weighing myself every morning made me worry less about my weight, and I could concentrate on achieving the other CBT-E goals.

In summary

In-session collaborative weighing consists of weekly weighing and recording, and personalised education about weight and weighing. It has five main goals:

1. To correct your misconceptions about weight changes
2. To provide reliable information about your weight

3. To help you to interpret the number on the scales correctly
4. To address frequent weight checking and/or weight avoidance
5. To reduce your weight concerns

• Take-home message

Through collaborative weighing, you will learn to interpret your weight scientifically and therefore overcome your irrational fears.

11

The Eating Problem Check List (EPCL)

The Eating Problem Check List, the EPCL for short, is a questionnaire designed to help you monitor the status of your eating disorder on a week-by-week basis. It is easy to complete and contains 16 questions on the main behaviours and concerns typically reported by people with eating disorders.

Once a week, immediately after the collaborative weighting and the review of your monitoring records, your therapist will ask you to fill in the EPCL to evaluate how things have gone over the last week. To make sure that the information you put on the EPCL is accurate, you should refer to your monitoring records for the previous seven days.

You should complete the EPCL truthfully and accurately, because your responses will help you and your therapist to assess the progress you have made and any obstacles you may have encountered during the week.

After you have completed the EPCL, together with your therapist you will fill in the "EPCL score summary sheet," which is designed to monitor your progress week by week by keeping a tally of your weekly weight and EPCL scores. Discussing your EPCL score summary sheet with your therapist, together with a collaborative review of your monitoring records for the week, will help you to see the changes you have made in the various behavioural and psychological expressions of your eating disorder. Understanding how the modification of certain behaviours (e.g., by adopting regular eating, reducing dietary restraint, weekly weighing and/or interrupting dysfunctional body checking) is associated with a reduction in concerns about eating, shape and weight over time—one of the primary goals of CBT-E.

Furthermore, highlighting the expressions of your eating disorder that you need to address will enable you and your therapist to focus on specific manifestations of your eating disorder, and therefore guide your treatment.

You can find a blank EPCL (Table 28.4) and EPCL score summary sheet (Table 28.5) in the CBT-E tools at the back of this book. Your therapist will

DOI: 10.4324/9781003342489-13

Table 11.1 The Eating Problem Check List (EPCL) 3.1

INSTRUCTIONS: The following questions are concerned with the past seven days only. Please read each question carefully. Please answer all the questions. Thank you.

In the past seven days . . . *(indicate the number of times that this has occurred in the box on the right)*	**No. of episodes**
Have I eaten a large amount of food with a sense of having lost control (i.e., an objective binge-eating episode)?	
Have I eaten a not large amount of food with a sense of having lost control (i.e., a subjective binge-eating episode)?	
Have I made myself sick (vomited) as a means of controlling my shape and weight?	
Have I taken laxatives as a means of controlling my shape and weight?	
Have I taken diuretics (water pills) as a means of controlling my shape and weight?	
Have I exercised excessively as a means of controlling my weight, shape or amount of fat, or to burn? extra calories.	
Have I weighed myself?	

In the past seven days . . . *(tick which box is true for you)*	**0 Never**	**1 Rarely**	**2 Sometimes**	**3 Often**	**4 Always**
Have I avoided some foods as a means of controlling my weight, shape and/or eating?					
Have I reduced my food portions as a means of controlling my weight, shape and/or eating?					
Have I checked my food (e.g., calorie counting, weighing food, checking the food's nutritional content)?					
Have I checked my shape (e.g., looking at parts of my body in the mirror; measuring the circumference of parts of my body; compared my body shape with that of other people)?					
Have I avoided my body (e.g., avoided weighing, avoided particular clothes, avoided looking at my body)?					

Table 11.1 (Continued)

In the past seven days . . . *(tick which box is true for you)*	**0 Never**	**1 Rarely**	**2 Sometimes**	**3 Often**	**4 Always**
Have I felt fat?					
Have I been preoccupied with my weight?					
Have I been preoccupied with my shape?					
Have I been preoccupied with my eating control?					

Source: Adapted with permission from Dalle Grave, R., Sartirana, M., Milanese, C., El Ghoch, M., Brocco, C., Pellicone, C., & Calugi, S. (2019). Validity and reliability of the Eating Problem Checklist. *Eating Disorders*, *27*(4), 384–399. doi:10.1080/10640266.2018.1528084

provide you with a copy of two tools. However, you can photocopy them in this book or download them using the QR code:

EPCL

EPCL score summary sheet

In summary

The Eating Problem Check List (EPCL) is a 16-item questionnaire designed to assess your eating-disorder behaviours and concerns session by session. You should fill it in once a week after a joint review of your monitoring records with your therapist.

You should fill in the EPCL truthfully and accurately because your responses will tell you and your therapist how you are doing and any obstacles you encounter each week. This assessment can then be used to update your personal formulation and highlight any issues that need to be addressed.

• Take-home message

The EPCL is a good indicator of your progress towards all your CBT-E goals. It provides a weekly snapshot of how far you have come and where you need to go next.

Establishing regular eating

Establishing a regular eating pattern is the foundation for building other changes. It focuses on your eating patterns—*when* to eat rather than what or how much to eat. The goal is to eat three planned meals and two or three snacks at regular intervals throughout the day.

This procedure is of enormous benefit to people whose eating patterns are disrupted, because they binge eat and/or because they restrict their diet. If you experience binge-eating episodes, establishing regular eating rapidly reduces the frequency of this behaviour. This is generally accompanied by a marked improvement in mood as you realise that it *is* possible for you to take control over your eating. That is why the regular eating procedure is introduced in Step One—any residual binge-eating episodes that remain are addressed during Step Two.

Regular eating produces a reduction in binge eating through the following mechanisms:

1. It provides structure and control if you have dysregulated eating habits, like "grazing" instead of eating defined meals and snacks.
2. If you have high levels of dietary restraint, it tackles infrequent or delayed eating.
3. If you are low weight, it is better (and less threatening) to establish a pattern of regular eating before you start thinking about eating more. The main reasons for this are the following:

    - You need to eat regular meals and snacks before portion size can be increased.
    - Regular eating is a change that is not too hard to accomplish since it does not involve increasing what is eaten.
    - Regular eating tackles the tendency to delay eating—a form of dieting frequently adopted by low-weight people with eating disorders.
    - It seems to lessen the propensity to feel full.
    - After a few weeks, it generally reduces the degree of preoccupation with food and eating.

DOI: 10.4324/9781003342489-14

The procedure

There are two elements to the intervention:

1. Eating at regular, scheduled intervals throughout the day
2. Not eating in between

Eating at regular intervals throughout the day

This involves adopting an eating pattern comprising three planned meals each day, plus two or three planned snacks. For example:

- Breakfast
- Mid-morning snack
- Lunch
- Mid-afternoon snack
- Evening meal
- Evening snack (if appropriate)

Here are some suggestions to help you get the most out of the regular eating procedure:

Give priority to regular eating

Eating at the planned times should take precedence over other daily activities. You must stick to the timetable, whatever your appetite. However, you can adjust your eating schedule to suit your day-to-day commitments. For instance, you can eat at different times on school/work days and days off.

Plan ahead

You should always know when you will be having your next meal or snack and what it will be. If your therapist calls you out of the blue, you should be able to tell them when and what you will be eating next. Each morning (or the evening before), you should write out an outline of the plan for the day at the top of the day's monitoring record. If you don't know exactly what will be happening that day, make a rough estimate and identify a time when you will take stock and plan the remainder of the day.

Do not leave more than a four-hour gap between planned meals and snacks, and do not skip any of them

Remember that the consequences of skipping or delaying a meal or a snack are an increased risk of overeating or binge-eating later on, as well as greater preoccupation with food and eating, and perpetuating the tendency to feel full. Every meal you skip feeds the cycle.

Choose what to eat in your meals and snacks

In Step One, regular eating is focused only on planning mealtimes and sticking to the plan. If you don't know what to eat, try to adopt a varied and flexible diet. Try to eat your five food groups and avoid compensatory behaviour, such as vomiting, spitting or laxative misuse. Purging after meals or snacks is against the rules. You are also firmly discouraged from calorie counting, especially keeping a running total.

Eat at normal times, not when your eating disorder dictates

Most people eat at set times or together with others, regardless of whether or not they are hungry. Stick to your planned mealtimes, whether you feel hungry or full. Remember that your eating disorder has almost certainly disturbed your perception of hunger. Once you have been eating regularly (without purging) for several months, your hunger and fullness signalling will return to normal. Even then, though, it is better not to rely exclusively on these sensations as indicators of when to eat.

Carefully plan social eating

For instance, if the choice of what to eat is likely to be limited (as at a dinner party at a friend's house) or vast (at a buffet), you should have a look what food is available and take a little time out for planning. Go into another room for a minute to decide what you are going to eat and how to stick to your regular eating pattern. If you are at risk of overeating, put down your cutlery and plate as soon as you have finished what you planned.

If your eating habits are chaotic or highly restrictive, you can introduce regular eating patterns in steps

You could, for example, introduce regular eating to the part of the day when your eating causes the fewest problems, usually in the mornings. Once you have mastered this part of the day, you can focus on another section of the day, and so on, until you establish a regular eating pattern spanning the entire day.

Evening snacks are important if you are prone to evening binges

For obvious reasons, if this applies to you, it is essential that you include an evening snack in your regular eating plan.

Not eating between meals and snacks

If you find it difficult to resist eating between planned meals and snacks, a procedure we call "things to say and things to do" may help. This procedure is especially useful if you are prone to binge-eating episodes, or if you tend to eat many small meals throughout the day. When you are faced with a strong urge to eat, you should distract yourself, step out of the moment by doing or saying something you have prepared earlier.

Things to do

This involves doing something to take your mind off food, an activity that makes binge eating less likely. This needs to be done for 1–2 hours at most, by which time the urge to eat is likely to have waned and, in any case, you will be due to eat. You need to be ready to act as soon as the urge to eat comes upon you, so before you start you should create a list of suitable activities, or "things to do" to have on hand. Possible activities incompatible with eating are:

- Interpersonal activities like chatting, phoning or visiting friends
- Getting out of the situation by going outside for a walk, for example
- Changing the atmosphere by playing music that makes you want to dance or sing rather than eat

Things to say

This strategy is also known as "urge surfing"—you take a moment to ride out the urge to eat until it wanes. Your "things to say" should be phrases that make it easier for you to tolerate the urge. Once again, you should prepare what you are going to say—your own personal mantra—beforehand. For example, you might say something like this:

- "I CAN tolerate this urge without bingeing."
- "The urge to binge is like a wave—it increases until it reaches a peak, and then wears off. I'm going to wait it out."
- "I'm not hungry, I just feel a little anxious/sad/nervous/bored (as applicable). I'm not going to binge."

You should take deep, slow breaths and think about the urge dispassionately rather than trying to make it go away. The more you do this, the more quickly you learn to decentre from the urge so it no longer controls your eating. You will find that eventually the urge generally dissipates within a few minutes. If it takes longer, you should resort to your list of things to do.

While the things to do can be used in the early stages of treatment, the things to say tends to be less effective, at least in the beginning. We therefore suggest using them when your urges to eat between meals and snacks are intermittent and less overwhelming. To help you remember how you have decided to handle these situations, you might find it helpful to write your things to say and do down on a "coping card," which you can keep close by for when you need it.

Figure 12.1 shows an example monitoring record filled in by Monica, who is applying the regular eating procedure. As you can see, she planned ahead ("Today's plan") when, what and where to eat, using the first three columns of the monitoring record. Then, underneath, she used the same sheet to monitor her eating in real time, indicating any transgressions and why they occurred

Day Monday **Date** 6th September

Time	Food and drink	Place	*	V/L/E	Context and comments
	Today's plan				
7:00	I cup of skimmed milk with cereals	Kitchen			
10:30	I apple	School			
13:30	Salad with tuna	Kitchen			
16:30	I yogurt	Kitchen			
19:30	Turkey with rice and spinach	Kitchen			
	I yogurt				
7:00	I cup of skimmed milk with cereal }	Kitchen			Ok
10:30	I apple	School			
13:30	Salad with tuna	Kitchen			
	6 almonds		*		They were on the table. I couldn't resist
	2 glasses of still water				
14:30	I chocolate bar	Kitchen	*		I shouldn't have eaten this chocolate bar but I was tired.
16:30			E		I skipped this snack because I had already eaten a chocolate bar. I walked for 60 minutes to burn off the calories.
19:30	Turkey with rice and spinach	Kitchen			I didn't have the yogurt. I've already eaten enough today.
	2 glasses of still water				

Figure 12.1 An example monitoring record filled in by Monica, who is working on applying the regular eating procedure

Common difficulties with regular eating

Here we describe the most common difficulties that people with eating disorders say they have in establishing a regular eating pattern, and some advice on overcoming them.

> *Knowing in advance what I'm going to eat increases my concern about eating. I want to be free and more spontaneous.*

In this event, you should think about whether you feel free and spontaneous when you don't plan ahead. Were your difficulties eating regular meals and snacks brought on by your concern about the effect of eating on your shape and weight? If this is the case, remember that the regular eating procedure will provide you with information on the relationship between eating and weight, which can reduce concerns about both. In any event, you should consider regular eating as temporary, as the ultimate goal of the therapy is to help you become more spontaneous and eat freely. However, this will only be possible when your concerns about eating have been reduced.

> *I have* never *eaten five times per day, and neither do my family or friends.*

If you have this objection, try to consider the regular pattern of eating a kind of medicine schedule—a key procedure to overcoming your eating disorder. Remember that it is only temporary—once you are recovered, you will be able to eat when you want. However, while treatment is underway, it is in your best interests to stick to a regular eating plan. In addition, eating regular meals and snacks is healthy.

> *I don't want to eat so many meals and snacks; it'll make me put on weight.*

This seldom happens, as nobody is asking you to change what or how much you eat. If you have binge-eating episodes, regular eating reduces binge-eating frequency and will therefore significantly decrease your energy intake. As we have seen, you absorb a significant number of calories through bingeing, even if you purge.

> *I feel full even after eating relatively little.*

That is fine, as at this stage you can eat as much or as little as you like, just as long as you eat what you planned, when you planned it. We know that feeling full is especially strong if you are low weight, as chronic undereating slows your digestion. However, this feeling generally subsides within an hour, and once a regular eating pattern is in place, your feeling full will gradually decline.

Planning in advance does not work; when I don't stick to my eating plan, I binge.

This is a dangerous example of all-or-nothing thinking. Do you look on even a small deviation from your eating plan as a failure? Do you think it ruins the whole day? If so, think again. It's not the end of the world, and one small lapse should not sabotage your efforts thus far. Cry or shout if you need to, then take a few deep breaths, mentally turn over a new leaf and re-commit to your plan for the rest of the day. If this continues to be a problem for you, instead of "good days" and "bad days," try rating each day's compliance on a scale of 0 to 5.

Distraction activities are a waste of time.

It is not true that putting off eating will only delay the inevitable binge. Successfully surfing or distracting yourself from an urge to binge is a great achievement. It is not diminished by further urges to eat later in the day. Instead of focusing on daily goals, work from hour to hour using urge surfing and/or distraction activities between set meals and snacks to establish a stable eating pattern. Remember to keep your "coping card" at hand and consult it whenever you feel the urge.

Samantha's story

I've got a big family and mealtimes can be hectic in my house, but they are always an important part of the day. My problems with eating started when I was in middle school, when some girls started calling me fat. That really hurt so I talked to my paediatrician about it and she put me on a diet. My grandmother, who did the cooking, couldn't understand why I had to be given "rabbit food," rather than what everyone else was eating, and would grumble about it every day. This made mealtimes difficult, and my brothers started teasing me about what I was eating. I figured that the quicker I could lose the weight I needed to, the faster everything would go back to normal, so I got really serious about counting calories and not eating anything fattening. Well, I ended up losing 20 kg in about six months, and suddenly I was "too skinny" and had to go to therapy.

I didn't want to talk about my problems to my CBT-E therapist at first. I told her that I couldn't eat any more because I felt full as soon as I ate even the smallest mouthful. Eventually though I broke down and told her how lonely I felt and how annoyed my family made me, especially at mealtimes. I think on some level I realised that I needed help because I had started to binge eat. I was very scared of putting on weight and going right back to where I was before I started dieting.

However, I couldn't understand why I needed to eat two snacks a day. Nobody in my family eats snacks—there's plenty for everyone on the table at mealtimes. But then my therapist explained to me that regular eating would help me reduce my binge-eating episodes. She showed me, with the help of my formulation and monitoring records, that dividing the day up with three meals and two snacks would make it easier for me not to binge in between. She also promised me that eating regularly would help my digestion work properly, and stop me feeling full so quickly. I wasn't totally convinced that this would work, but even during the first week I started to feel better, and didn't binge once!

In summary

Eating regularly is the foundation on which other changes are built. The benefits of regular eating are:

- Providing structure to eating habits and the day
- Addressing skipping or delaying meals—one of the three forms of strict dieting (the other two are eliminating certain foods and reducing portions)
- Interrupting the cycle of binge-eating and dietary restriction

If you are low weight, it can also help to improve your digestion and reduce your early sense of fullness.

To eat regularly, it is necessary to do two things:

1. *Eat at regular, planned intervals throughout the day.* You will need to plan three meals plus two or three snacks in advance to be eaten at set times. It doesn't matter how much you eat, just what and when. Do not skip any meals or snacks, and don't go more than four hours without eating.
2. *Do not eat between planned meals and snacks.* If you feel the urge to eat between the times you have planned, use the urge surfing strategy or do something to distract you until either the urge subsides or it's time for the next meal or snack.

• Take-home message

Always know when and what you will be eating for your next meal or snack, and keep your list of things to do and/or list of things to say on hand.

13

Deciding to make the change

The first part of Step One has been designed to help you understand the psychological mechanisms maintaining your eating disorder. This puts you in a better position to decide to change or not to change. In the second part of Step One, you will discuss the implications of change with your therapist over the course of a few sessions (often three or more).

If you are underweight, the most important decision to change will be the decision to restore weight. This is also important if you have lost a significant amount of weight, even if your weight remains within the normal range. Indeed, this is indicative of atypical anorexia nervosa, which often has the same negative consequences as being underweight.

At the end of CBT-E Step One it is you who decides to regain weight, rather than having this decision imposed upon you. Undoubtedly, weight restoration will completely change your life for the better. The question is how to reach this important but challenging decision. We find that the best way is to think carefully about how your eating disorder is affecting you now, and how it will continue to affect you down the line. Is that really how you want your life to be? Or would you prefer a happier, healthier future? CBT-E can help you make the decision. Read on to find out how.

Why do I need to regain weight?

There are five main reasons to work towards regaining weight if you have a low weight:

1. *To reverse starvation symptoms*. Some adverse effects of your eating disorder are a direct result of being significantly low weight. By regaining the weight, you will make them disappear for good. For example:
    - Preoccupation with food and eating
    - Being inflexible, having to stick to routines and/or inability to be spontaneous

DOI: 10.4324/9781003342489-15

- Having difficulty making decisions
- Not wanting to socialise
- Having difficulty concentrating
- Sleeping poorly
- Feeling full quickly
- Feeling very cold
- Feeling physically weak

2. *To find your true personality.* How you feel now—lonely, tired and insecure—is not who you really are. It is the consequence of being underweight. Can you remember how you were before the eating disorder? Once you have regained weight you will return to your cheerful, charming self.
3. *To prevent lasting physical harm.* Several of the physical consequences of being such a low weight are life-changing and/or life-threatening. They cause long-term damage to your health, particularly your bones and heart, and may even kill you.
4. *To break the chains of your eating disorder.* Some of the effects of being underweight are maintaining your eating disorder. The effects of being low weight intensify the overvaluation of shape and weight and your need for control over eating through several mechanisms. Have a look at Monica's formulation in Figure 13.1 as an example. As you can see, Monica doesn't think that low weight and strict dieting are a problem. However, by making her feel proud of herself for achieving them, what they are actually doing is increasing the importance she gives to them—they are making that slice of the pie even bigger. Worrying about food all the time does the same

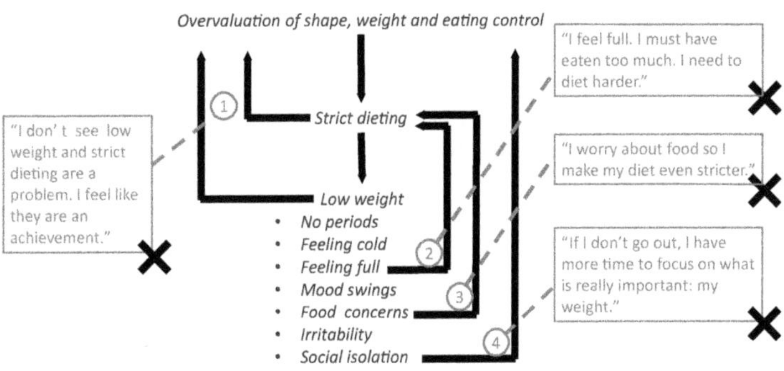

Figure 13.1 An example personal formulation drawn up by Monica, an underweight young person with an eating disorder, highlighting how her misconceptions and the effects of significantly low weight act to maintain her eating disorder

thing and makes her even more determined to lose weight. Feeling full also makes her step up her efforts to diet, because she takes it as a signal that she has eaten too much, although we have seen that, in reality, feeling full is a starvation symptom. Last but not least, the social withdrawal caused by her eating disorder actually intensifies it by preventing her from having experiences that reduce the importance she gives to shape, weight and eating control.

More information on the effect of low weight and starvation symptoms is described in Chapter 3 and summarised in Table 3.1. All these effects of low weight will disappear when your weight returns to normal.

Deciding to change

As you discuss the decision to change, your therapist will ask you to:

1. Focus on the present by creating a current pros-and-cons-of-change table (in one session)
2. Focus on the future by creating a future pros-and-cons-of-change table (in the next session)
3. Draw conclusions and write them down
4. "Take the plunge"

The present

Your therapist will ask you to consider your reasons for and against change. What advantages and disadvantages are there to overcoming your eating disorder? If you are underweight, the change will require that you regain weight. You need to get above the minimum BMI threshold of 19 or the corresponding BMI-for-age percentile if you are under 16, as this is generally the minimum weight needed to be free from the adverse effects of being underweight.

We find it is best to first discuss why you *do not* want to change or are afraid to do so. These will include the positive things that you think being low weight brings to your life that you are afraid of losing. Write these reasons down on the left side of a sheet of paper under the heading REASONS TO STAY AS I AM. This will be your *current pros-and-cons-of-change table.*

Once you have listed the "cons" of change, you should shift your focus to your reasons for taking the opportunity to change. Think about all the adverse effects of your eating disorder on all aspects of your life, including relationships with others (parents, friends, etc.), your physical and psychological wellbeing, school performance and ability to engage in other valued activities. Write these on the right side of the paper, under the heading REASONS TO MAKE THE CHANGE.

Table 13.1 Julia's current pros and cons of change

Reasons to stay as I am	*Reasons to make the change*
I feel in control. *I like to be thin and sometimes that makes me feel beautiful.* *If I change:* • *I will not be so thin.* • *Others will think I am getting fat.* • *Others will think that I eat too much.* • *My legs, hips, arms, stomach and face will get fat again.* • *I will not be able to fit in all my clothes.* • *I will be envious of girls that are thinner than me.*	*I would not be tired and would sleep better.* *I would stop being cold.* *I would be able to take up sport again.* *I would be less unhappy.* *I would be able to go out to eat with my friends.* *I would be less obsessed with food.* *My parents would be less sad and angry with me.*

Remember that it is normal to be in two minds about change. You should not expect to have a eureka moment and "see the light" at this stage. However, you will get a balanced, objective understanding of what your eating disorder gives you, and what it takes away, as in the example drawn up by Julia shown in Table 13.1.

You will prepare your *current pros-and-cons-of-change table* during one session with your therapist. Then you should take home a copy and reflect upon it before the next session, when you will review it together.

The future

After reviewing your current pros-and-cons-of-change table with your therapist, you will begin to discuss your future. Think about what your life will be like in six months to a year. Consider how the eating disorder would affect your plans and aspirations. The following questions may help you think more clearly:

> *Imagine having a time machine and the possibility to travel to a not-too-distant future—for example, six months or one year ahead. What do you imagine that your life will be like? Do you have any plans for the future? What are they?*

> *How would you like to spend the summer? With whom? Would you like to go on holiday? What would that be like?*

> *What about school? What about your relationships with your classmates and teachers? Would you like to go on a school trip? Do you feel that you would be able to go? What about your exams at the end of high school? What about going to college?*

Table 13.2 Julia's pros of change, when thinking about her future (in one year's time)

Reasons to make the change
I want to be free. *I want to finish the school year.* *I want to go out with my friends and to parties.* *I want to eat without anxiety and fear.* *I don't want to be tired and cold or have dry skin.* *I want to be physically fit.* *I want to take up doing sport again.* *I want my parents to be happy and not sad for me.* *I want to be a cheerful person like I was before the eating disorder.*

Would you like to have interests outside of school? If so, what would you like to do?

What sort of relationships would you like to have with other people? What about friends and social life? What about relationships with your family? What about romantic relationships?

What sort of person would you like to be? How would you like to feel about yourself? What sort of values would you like to have? What would you like to be important to you?

Do you think that staying this way might interfere with these things?

Finally, write your ideas down in a *future pros-and-cons-of-change table* in session with your therapist. Take home a copy, mull it over and modify it if you want. Then, take it to the next session, when you will review it with your therapist.

An example of the pros section of a future pros-and-cons-of-change table, once again drawn up by Julia, is shown in Table 13.2.

Drawing conclusions

The next step involves a detailed point-by-point discussion with your therapist about what you wrote in your current and future pro-and-cons-of-change tables. During this discussion, you should focus on the likely impact of not taking the opportunity to change. How will this affect your aspirations? Do not underestimate your reasons *for* change, as the benefits of no longer being low weight and overcoming the eating disorder cannot be understated.

You should also explore in detail your reasons for *not* wanting to change. Weigh them up against your reasons for change. Are they as vital as you

Table 13.3 Julia's conclusion table

Conclusions
I want to get better and regain weight because: • *I will be healthier. I will not be tired and will sleep better. I will stop being cold. My periods will come back.* • *I will be happier and a cheerful person like I was before the eating disorder.* • *I will be less obsessed with food.* • *I will be able to take up sport again.* • *I will be able to go out to eat with my friends.* • *I will finish the school year.* • *My parents will be less sad with me.* • *I will become physically fit. I will not become fat.* • *I will eat without anxiety and fear, and I will be able to have true control of my eating. This will protect me from overeating and gaining weight without control.*

thought? We often find that when they are written down, reasons not to change do not seem so important in the big scheme of things. They are often short-term barriers that ordinarily you would not allow to condition your life. Remember that this is the effect of your eating disorder. Maintaining a persistent low weight will prevent you developing a healthy, balanced self-evaluation system—the main goal you are aiming for by regaining control of your eating, shape and weight.

Know too that your eating disorder is highly unlikely to disappear unless you do something about it. If you don't decide to change, your maintenance mechanisms will remain in place and you may even develop new ones. Remember that your eating disorder is likely to migrate, and six months down the line you may find yourself binge eating and gaining weight uncontrollably. Indeed, up to two-thirds of underweight people with an eating disorder start binge eating, and up to a half develop typical bulimia nervosa. Considered this information, and remind yourself of your plans and hopes for the future. How would they be affected if you still had an eating disorder?

The exploration and examination of your reasons not to change should not be hurried and, in some cases, may take a few sessions. Between these sessions, think about what you have discussed and write down any further concerns or questions you may have for when you next see your therapist. When you are ready, your therapist will help you draw up a *conclusions table* (see Julia's example in Table 13.3).

Taking the plunge

> *The sooner you start, the sooner you will experience the benefits of change; putting it off just prolongs the agony and increases the risk of you having long-standing problems. It's like standing at the edge of a swimming pool and delaying diving in*

because the water looks cold and uninviting. It's better just to take the plunge. Shall we begin?

After having dedicated a few sessions to weighing up the pros and cons of change, if you are still undecided what to do, we suggest telling yourself something like this: "It's time to take the plunge and start addressing change. The sooner I start, the sooner I will begin to feel the benefits of change."

If necessary, you can consider the change as an experiment. Remind yourself that if you do not like its effects, you can easily return to your old way of living after the treatment ends. This would not be difficult—indeed, it would be all too easy. However, in our long clinical experience, we have not encountered any patient who has chosen to do this. Instead, patients tend to say that they wish they had changed sooner because their life is so much better than it was.

It is important to note that it is natural for motivation to change to wax and wane and will therefore be an ongoing issue in treatment. Your motivation may need to be addressed several times. However, if you feel your resolve slipping, all you have to do is bring it up with your therapist, who will be able to help you out. But that is for the future; let us focus on now: think about the special opportunity you have to improve your life. Don't you want to take the plunge?

If you decide not to address weight restoration at the end of this process, the therapist will likely refer you for a different form of treatment. Remember that to succeed, CBT-E needs you to be in the driving seat. If you are unwilling to start the engine, you are not going to get very far.

Rebecca's story

I've always been crazy about dancing. I started when I was really young, and I was really good at it for a while. Then, when I was 16, I began to get the impression that my dance teacher wasn't as pleased with me as she used to be. In my eyes, she was more impressed with the other students, who were all thinner than me. I thought that if I could lose some weight, my dancing would improve and I could go back to being top of the class, so I asked my mother (she's divorced and I only see my father every other weekend) if I could see a nutritionist. He gave me a diet to follow, which I did for a while, but then there was a big dance audition coming up. I was really anxious about it, especially because I felt that I wasn't as good as the other girls, so I started restricting my diet even more. This made me feel better for a while—I thought I was taking control of the situation. However, rather than my dance routine, my mind was filled with thoughts about food and my "wobbly bits," and I began to stress about that too. Both of my parents began to worry about my health and started to push me into eating more. They tried to bring it home to me that if I weighed too little, I wouldn't be able to pursue my dreams of a dancing career. I tried to eat more, I really did, but that made me feel like I was losing control, so if I felt I'd ate too much, I'd just skip the next meal. This meant I lost even more weight, and ended up at a BMI of 16.1. My periods had stopped by this point, too.

I realised that my parents were right, and that something needed to be done, so I did a bit of research on the internet. I liked the idea of CBT-E, because it put me, rather than the doctors, in control of my own recovery, so I signed up for therapy. I told my therapist about my dietary rules, and the fact that I always felt cold, weak, lonely, moody and anxious, and that I was always thinking about food. She explained to me that these were symptoms of something called "starvation syndrome" and entirely caused by my not eating enough. She didn't seem judgemental about this, though, which made it a lot easier for me to open up to her in a way that I hadn't been able to with my parents or my dance coach. Because she was so understanding, I told her how afraid I was of gaining weight—my entire career was at stake! She asked me whether I was more concerned about gaining weight or passing the audition, and I have to admit I found that difficult to answer. This helped me understand that I did place too much value on my shape and weight, and I agreed to commit myself to the tasks in Step One.

Once I'd started therapy, I found out I'd passed the audition and got into the dance academy. However, that was in another city and I had to continue CBT-E remotely. Moving away was a big change, and I was a little anxious and down. I was having trouble sleeping and I was terrified that I wouldn't be able to keep up in class. Being kicked out of dance academy would really make me feel like a failure. It would be the death of a dream that I had had since I could remember. This made me determined to succeed at CBT-E, but I was still worried about having to put on weight. My parents were worried about this too. They told my therapist that they thought the CBT-E goal of reaching a normal weight would be incompatible with dancing. However, after a bit of discussion, both they and I decided that it would be best to put my health first.

It was a big decision to start weight restoration, but my therapist didn't ask me to change overnight. We spent four sessions discussing how my eating disorder was affecting my life now, and how it would affect my life in the future. We drew up a table of my reasons for and against change, which made it easier for me to see why it was necessary to do so. I was sick of feeling trapped and different. I wanted to be carefree and to be able to concentrate on my dancing. I knew that if I wanted to be a good dancer, I would have to be in peak physical condition—not malnourished and underweight. I knew it would not be an easy road, but I really wanted to start Step Two. It was time I tackled weight restoration.

In summary

The second part of Step One is dedicated to evaluating the pros and cons of change and addressing weight regain (if applicable). The goal of CBT-E is that you decide to regain weight rather than having this decision forced upon you.

This process requires the application of the following steps across several consecutive sessions with your therapist:

1. Focusing on the present by creating a current pros-and-cons-of-change table
2. Focusing on the future by creating a future pros-and-cons-of-change table
3. Drawing conclusions
4. "Taking the plunge"

• Take-home message

Think about the things that your eating disorder gives you, and the things it takes (and will continue to take) away. What have you really got to lose by taking the plunge? What have you got to gain?

14

Involving your parents

Your parents may help you create an optimum family environment and, with your agreement, support you in implementing some treatment procedures.

CBT-E is a one-on-one treatment, but your parent(s) are always involved in the treatment if you are younger than 18, or with your consent if you are 18 years old or older. If you are of age and no longer live with your family of origin, significant others, like friends or a partner, may be influencing your eating. Hence, with your consent, it would be helpful to recruit their support. They could be invaluable in creating an environment for you that makes it easier for you to change. What we say about parents in this chapter is generally applicable to significant others, so read on to find out what they can do for you.

The most important way your parents can assist you on your CBT-E journey is to create a home environment that supports your efforts to change. You may also like to ask them to help you get to grips with some treatment procedures. Remember that your therapist is *your* therapist, and not a family counsellor or an agent of your parents. Parental involvement will therefore be limited to one parent-only session during the first week of treatment (if you are under 18) and joint sessions with you and your parents at the end of a few of your individual sessions. This means that your parents will not have the opportunity to hijack your treatment, compromising your ability to bring about your own recovery. You will be in the driving seat and will always have the final say. However, know that if you report any dangerous behaviour that puts your life at risk to your therapist, they have an ethical, professional and legal duty to disclose it to your parents.

If there are any reasons that you feel that recruiting your parents would not be helpful, make sure you discuss them with your therapist. Likewise, if your parents wish to disclose anything relevant to your therapist, they will be encouraged to do so during the joint sessions while you are present. They should not contact your therapist outside of this joint space.

DOI: 10.4324/9781003342489-16

Parent-only sessions

Your parents are seen alone only once, during the first week of the treatment. The topics that will be addressed with your parents during the parent-only session will be thoroughly explained to you by your therapist before the session. In general, though, this session is held so your therapist can educate your parents about your eating disorder, as envisioned by the psychological CBT-E model, and learn a little about your family environment. During this session, your therapist will look for factors that could help your parents create an optimal family environment for your recovery and identify anything that might hinder your efforts to get well—we call these *barriers to change*. This session is also an opportunity to address any distress your parents may feel about your eating disorders. Although entirely unwarranted, parents often blame themselves, and it may be helpful for yours to talk it through with your therapist if they feel this way.

As regards creating a supportive environment for your recovery, what your therapist suggests to your parents will vary from case to case but will likely include the following:

- *Adopt a warm and supportive communication style. Stop criticising eating behaviour* (if this is a problem in your family). Criticism will not help you to overcome the eating disorder. On the contrary, it will impact your mood, which may aggravate your eating-disorder behaviours. As we have seen, young people often try to get rid of negative moods through unhealthy coping strategies—for example, further dietary restraint, binge eating or other dysfunctional mood- modulation behaviours like self-harm and/or drug or alcohol misuse.
- *Spend stress-free time together*. Your parents will be encouraged to spend time with you in a peaceful and relaxed way in a supportive atmosphere. They will be asked to share enjoyable activities, relive happy memories and generally have fun together with you, away from food. These positive experiences and emotions can help distract you from your preoccupation with shape, weight and eating control and introduce balance and variety into your thinking and behaviours—a space in which your eating disorder does not hold sway.
- *Take time for themselves and ask for support*. The road to your recovery is usually long, and your parents will therefore be advised to pace themselves and take the journey one step at a time. They will be encouraged to have a support network in place for times of need and to dedicate time to self-care.
- *Ban dieting*. It is very difficult for a person with an eating disorder to tackle dietary restraint and restriction if another family member is on a weight-loss diet. So, if one of your parents or another family member is attempting to lose weight, for your sake they should stop while you are in treatment.

- *Ban fasting.* While it may be necessary for your parents to fast for religious reasons or give something up for Lent, CBT-E is impossible to implement while fasting. While you are undergoing treatment, therefore, fasting in the family might be detrimental to your recovery and should be avoided.
- *Tailor food stores.* If you have recurrent binge-eating episodes, your parents may be asked to keep highly processed/high-calorie foods to a minimum and out of sight at home. On the other hand, if you avoid certain foods and have planned to introduce them to your diet with the therapist, your parents may be asked to buy some specific foods for you.
- *Avoid conversational triggers.* Comments about your eating during meals (positive or negative) can trigger negative emotions that can adversely affect your eating. These include compliments or criticism about eating habits or food choices, whether directed at you or anybody else.
- *Create a "new" home environment.* Changing some simple family habits can convey the feeling of a fresh start. If the family does not eat together, we strongly recommended that your parents ensure that you start doing so now, because family meals can introduce healthy and protective habits. Your parents might also be asked to try adjusting the seating arrangements of family members at the table, buying new dishes, cups and/or cutlery, playing music during mealtimes and/or making minor changes to the layout at home. Things like too many mirrors, or books, magazines, and social media accounts focused on fitness, diet or the body and television shows devoted to dieting, cooking, and fashion can be unhelpful and disruptive to recovery from excessive body shape and weight concerns. Therefore, if possible, your parents should reduce the number of mirrors at home (to make frequent body checking difficult), get rid of books and magazines on diet and body-related topics and avoid watching triggering television shows that overly focus on cooking, baking, fashion or modelling, or glorify excessively thin, athletic or attractive actors.

Joint sessions

Some joint sessions with you and your parents will take place when the treatment is underway. The main goals of these joint sessions, typically held at the end of a one-to-one session with your therapist, are to keep your parents informed and involved in the treatment process and up to date on your progress. These sessions also discuss how your parents might help you by creating an optimal family environment, supporting your attempts to change and helping you implement some of the key treatment procedures.

The frequency and number of these sessions are not set in stone, and will be decided based on your evolving needs. In general, however, the first joint session with you and your parents will be held after the CBT-E regular eating procedure is introduced in Step One, usually in the second week of treatment. The therapist will use this session to explain to your parents precisely how they can help you.

Another joint session is usually scheduled one week later to review how regular eating is going and to address any issues you or your parents may have. Additional joint sessions may be scheduled when you have decided to tackle weight restoration (if applicable) to discuss the role of your parents before, during and after meals. Further joint sessions may be held as treatment progresses if you and your therapist think your parents' support in some CBT-E procedures might be beneficial.

As a general principle, CBT-E procedures are introduced and discussed with you first, and then with your parents. In a one-to-one session with you alone, your therapist will explain the CBT-E strategy in question, how it works and the practical aspects of implementing it. Then, if you agree to implement the strategy and believe that your parents would be in a position to help, your parents will be invited to join the session.

Some examples of the kind of help you can ask your parents for with specific CBT-E procedures are the following (refer to the relevant chapters for more information on the individual procedures):

- *Personal formulation*. Your parents are not involved in the drafting of your personal formulation. However, it is helpful that you explain it to them, with the therapist's help if you need it. This will allow them to understand the psychological nature of your eating disorder and the maintenance factors you are going to try to address.
- *Self-monitoring*. Your parents are advised not to read your monitoring records. Doing so is likely to negatively affect what and how you write and will therefore compromise the treatment's success.
- *Collaborative weighing*. As with the monitoring records, we recommend that your parents do not look at or comment on your weight chart.
- *Establishing regular eating*. Your parents can be very helpful in helping you to establish a pattern of regular eating. The extent of their involvement will depend on your needs, but some suggestions that the therapist commonly gives to parents are the following:
    - To let you be free to plan the foods you wish to eat for your meals and snacks, and to ensure that those foods are available at home
    - To work jointly with you to prepare your meals and snacks, following your written plan
    - To try to eat most meals with you, whenever possible
    - To create a positive atmosphere by avoiding discussions about food and not engaging in arguments during meals
    - To avoid pushing you to eat more than planned
    - To be supportive and not coercive
    - To help you practice distracting activities after eating to help you to control the urge to use compensatory behaviours

- *Deciding to gain weight.* It is almost inevitable that you will discuss the pros and cons of change and the attempt to tackle weight regain with your parents. However, remember that you are the expert here, and your discussions about the intricacies and complexities of the topic should be with your therapist, not your parents.
- *Tackling undereating and being low weight.* Essentially, your therapist will reiterate to your parents the importance of supporting you with your regular eating and explain the significance of working with you to choose and prepare family meals. Your parents will be encouraged to remain calm and supportive and to remind you to apply one or more of the psychological strategies (e.g., urge surfing) that have previously been discussed with your therapist if necessary.
- *Tackling dietary restraint.* Your parents will very likely be involved in helping you to address dietary restraint. For example, when you are working on overcoming food avoidance, they can accompany you to the supermarket to identify the foods you avoid. They can ensure that when you plan to eat an avoided food it is available, and they can accompany you to eat at a restaurant or café when you have agreed with your therapist to do so.
- *Tackling excessive exercising.* With your consent, your parents can be asked to help you limit excessive exercising and support you by doing distracting activities with you when you feel the urge to exercise.
- *Tackling overvaluation of shape and weight.* Your parents can help you to work on reducing the importance you attribute to weight and shape. For example, they may help and support you by removing unhelpful/excessive mirrors from the home, as well as any triggers of shape and weight concerns in the house (e.g., diet magazines). They will be taught about your body checking/avoidance and be asked to remind you how to stop it. They will also be asked to refrain from making comments about your or others' body weight or shape. Parents are usually the right people to help you overcome practical obstacles to expanding your interests (e.g., taking you to join a choir, setting up space at home for you to practice arts and crafts).
- *Dealing with events, moods, and eating.* Your parents can support your attempts to tolerate negative emotions and practice distracting activities. When they notice that you are getting into difficulty, they may also encourage you to use proactive problem-solving.
- *Tackling setbacks and mindset.* Your parents are informed on how the eating-disorder mindset works and why and how the mindset reactivation may occur. When this happens, they may engage you in distracting activities and remind you to use the problem-solving procedure you have learned.

A book to help them help you

Cognitive Behaviour Therapy for Eating Disorders in Young People. A Parents' Guide (Dalle Grave & el Khazen, 2002) is a book written specifically for parents (or significant others) of young people with an eating disorder undergoing CBT-E. The book is designed to provide helpful information on eating disorders and to suggest how they can support your recovery journey, and how not to get in your way. It includes up-to-date information on eating disorders and modern, innovative strategies and procedures for successfully involving them in your treatment as your "helpers," rather than your "controllers."

Your therapist will recommend that your parents read this book carefully. This will help them to better understand the psychological nature of your eating disorder, why you find it difficult to see dieting and low weight as a problem, why it is challenging for you to change and what they can do to lighten your load.

Susanne's story

As long as I can remember I've been a bit chubby, even though I've always done a lot of sport. I spent my entire teenage years on some diet or other, but I wasn't that bothered about my weight really, even when it started to go up during high school because I had to give up skateboarding and basketball—this was because I needed to study. In any case, there was nothing wrong with my life at that point. I never saw my father at all, but that was normal for me. My parents had been divorced since forever, and I got on really well with my mother's partner, who lived with us. My grades were good and I also thought I had a great relationship with my steady boyfriend. However, he dumped me in my last year of high school and started going out with another girl in my class. She was a lot thinner than me, and I got it into my head that he'd take me back if I was a skinny as she was. I went to see a nutritionist, who prescribed me a weight-loss diet. I also started exercising at home, doing sit-ups and stuff in study breaks, and I lost the weight I had set out to. At this point, my nutritionist said I should stop losing weight and gave me a weight-maintenance plan, but by now I'd already got the bug. I ignored their advice and started eating even less. I was exercising instead of studying, and my weight continued to drop. I had my first binge-eating episode in the summer. These got gradually more frequent, and I started putting on weight again. By Christmas I knew that things had really gone off the rails, so in the new year I started seen a psychiatrist and a psychotherapist. They helped me stop binge-eating, but I was still obsessed with eating control, and my body weight dropped to 48 kg.

Then I started university, and the binge-eating episodes came back. Because I started vomiting every time I binged, my weight didn't go up too much, but even at 55 kg I felt fat and really wanted to lose weight. I cut down even further on what I was eating and started purging after every meal. Because my weight got so low, I got admitted to a psychiatric inpatient unit for three weeks, which was dreadful. When I got out, my mother contacted a CBT-E clinic.

At the assessment session, they measured my weight as 40 kg. I admitted to my therapist that I thought about food constantly but was only eating one meal a day and exercising a lot, as well as making myself sick and taking laxatives on a daily basis. I told him that I was terrified of putting on weight and feeling really low and anxious. My periods had stopped a while back and I was weak and dizzy all the time. I told him that it would be difficult for me to try regular eating, because my mother tried to control everything I ate. She also followed me every time I went to the bathroom to try and stop me throwing up. I know it was because she was scared for me, but we would always end up arguing. To avoid this, I used to buy food in supermarkets and eat it there, which was humiliating. Taking laxatives also made me ashamed, because I had to hide it from her. My therapist discussed with me whether it might be a good idea to ask my mother to help. I wasn't thrilled with this idea, but he told me that together we could talk to my mother about giving me the space I needed to help me make the change. As I couldn't see any other way of getting her off my back, I agreed that we could have a joint session. I thought this might be stressful, but my therapist and I agreed to what we would talk about beforehand, which meant I felt more prepared. In the session itself, my therapist explained to my mother that my behaviour was under my control, and my control alone, and to get better it would be me that would have to change. He told her that to help me do this, I needed her to be a "supporter," not a "controller." It was a little upsetting to me to find out that my mother wasn't convinced that I could make the change by myself, but my therapist assured her that I had decided to do so, which was half the battle, and that if she continued to hound me, she would throw a spanner in the works. She agreed to give it a go, and in the long run I'm really grateful. It wasn't easy for her to bite her tongue because she was still really worried about me, but she gave me the space I needed and even helped me by doing my nails and other stuff after meals so it was easier for me to overcome the urge to run to the bathroom.

In summary

CBT-E is one-on-one treatment, and your therapist is YOUR therapist, not your parents'. However, it is helpful to involve your parents, and, with your consent, they will be asked to attend a parent-only session and a few joint sessions with you. In these sessions, they will be taught how to:

1. Create an optimal family environment that makes it easier for you to change
2. Help you implement some treatment procedures

As a general rule, CBT-E procedures are introduced and discussed with you first. Then, if you agree to implement the procedure and believe that your parents would be able to help, they will be invited to join the session to discuss what support they can offer.

• Take-home message

Although you will always be the one calling the shots, your parents can be helpful allies in the fight against your eating disorder.

Futhur Reading

Dalle Grave, R., & el Khazen, C. (2022). *Cognitive behaviour therapy for eating disorders in young people: A parents' guide*. London: Routledge.

15

Review sessions

The end of Step One, after three to four weeks, is a great time to take stock. In this review session you will discuss your progress with your therapist and make a plan for Step Two. A similar review will be scheduled every four weeks during Step Two if you need to work on regaining weight.

Reviewing your progress

Research on bulimia nervosa has shown that the more progress made during the first four weeks of treatment, the better the results at the end of treatment. So, the more control over your unhealthy weight-control behaviours you achieve in Step One, the more likely it is you will fully recover. This is why starting well is so important—it plants the seeds for later change. However, if things are not going so well, it is crucial to act quickly to find the causes and implement potential solutions. That is the primary purpose of this review session.

If you are not low weight, indicators that your treatment is progressing well are a reduction in the frequency of your binge-eating episodes (as a result of the regular eating procedure) and concerns about weight (as a result of the in-session weighing procedure). Your concerns about body shape will likely not have changed, because they have not yet been specifically addressed. If you are low weight, it is considered an improvement if you, after three to four weeks, agree to make the change and initiate weight regain after Step One, or if your weight increases by about 0.5 kg per week in Step Two.

You will discuss these improvements, and what helped you achieve them, with your therapist and then move on to identifying which problems remain and need to be addressed in the following sessions. If there have been problems, you will work on overcoming them by identifying any barriers to change.

Identifying barriers to change

If the treatment isn't working as well as expected, it is important to find out why so you can get back on the right track. The best way to do this is to find

DOI: 10.4324/9781003342489-17

out what is holding you back. This is why your therapist will want to talk to you about the following two points:

1. *Your attitude toward treatment*. Are you happy with the treatment? Do you consider the treatment suitable for you? What do you like/find difficult about it?
2. *Your use of the CBT-E procedures*. Which treatment procedures have you tried to use? How successful have they been? Why/why not?

Your personal formulation can also help you and your therapist identify your barriers to change. The following are some that we see most frequently,

Poor implementation of programme strategies and procedures

Ask yourself the following questions:

- Have you attended all the sessions?
- Have you been on time to all the sessions?
- Have you made your treatment a priority?
- Have you played an active role in your treatment?
- Have you monitored all your eating, events, thoughts and emotions influencing eating in real time?
- Have you weighed yourself only once a week in the session?
- Do you interpret your weight properly, or only focus on the number on the scales?
- Have you adopted the regular eating procedure?
- Have you planned your meals as suggested (if applicable)?

If you have not applied these strategies and procedures accurately because you have underestimated their importance, before deciding that the treatment doesn't work, have another go. Redouble your efforts and try to focus on getting it right. The programme does work, but you need to make it work.

Fear of no longer being "special" without the eating disorder

If this is true for you, you should analyse with your therapist what meaning you attach to "being special." Is it a way to get attention from other people? If so, try to think of healthier ways to attract attention from others. Is it *really* special to have an eating disorder? Carefully reread Chapters 3 and 4 and think about the psychological and physical features of your eating disorder. What is so special about thinking about food all day, being depressed or irritable, having no friends, not studying, being totally dependent on your parents and having the fitness level of an 80-year-old person and fragile bones?

Afraid of not knowing who you will be without the eating disorder

As described in Chapter 3, the effects of being low weight and undereating dramatically change who you are. Due to starvation symptoms, all people who don't eat enough have a very similar personality. In other words, being low weight and undereating makes you lose your uniqueness as a person. Getting out of the eating-disorder mindset will allow you to regain your authentic and unique personality. Do you want to be defined by your eating disorder? Is that really all you are?

Fear of no longer feeling in control without the eating disorder

Try to assess with your therapist whether you're really in control or not. Being in control means being able to relax your extreme dietary rules and other unhealthy weight-control behaviours for a few days without going into meltdown. Are you able to do that? If you can't, it means you don't have control of your eating. If you follow the programme, however, you will achieve real, healthy and flexible control of your diet.

Fear of no longer having an excuse to avoid scary things

Why do you need an excuse? Are you afraid of not being able to meet people's expectations? Is that really a good reason for remaining this way? Why does this excuse make it difficult for you to get to grips with your eating disorder? If you dedicated as much time and energy to something other than your shape and weight, don't you think you would excel at that?

Fear of being seen as weak if you put on weight

Are you sure that others will think you are weak if you recover from your eating disorder? The reverse is probably true. It is you who thinks that dieting makes you strong, but others admire people who are happy and confident in their own skin, despite the social pressure to look a certain way. They may, in fact, consider people with eating disorders superficial, weak and lacking self-control. In their minds, unconditioned by the eating-disorder mindset, it is strong people who overcome eating disorders.

Fear of losing control of eating and continuing to gain weight

This is a common fear of people with an eating disorder. However, the research indicates that people in remission from an eating disorder tend to maintain a low normal weight and healthy control of their diet. In contrast, strict dieting and maintaining a low body weight over a long period time of makes it more likely that you will binge eat, leading to gradual and uncontrolled weight gain. In other words, overcoming the eating disorder is the best strategy for maintaining long-term healthy weight control.

Inflexibility and difficulty in changing in general

Some people with eating disorders have problems making changes in general, not only in their eating behaviour. This difficulty is typical of people who also have clinical perfectionism. They are plagued by an underlying fear that they will not be able to master any changes in their routine. Low weight and under-eating often accentuate this problem, increasing indecision, inflexibility and the tendency to procrastinate. If rigidity and difficulty changing are problems that affect you, set aside your doubts for the time being. Take the plunge to attempt something that will change your life for the better. Wouldn't it be nice to live new life, no longer conditioned by the eating disorder? What have you really got to lose?

Clinical depression

Low mood is common in people with an eating disorder. It is mainly the consequence of low body weight, binge-eating episodes and/or the effect of the disorder on your quality of life—social isolation makes you miserable. This form of depression, called "secondary depression," is not treated by your therapist. This is because it does not create an obstacle to treatment and will go away on its own once you go into remission. However, if you have clinical depression, which is not brought on by your eating disorder, it may be interfering with your treatment. Clinical depression interacts negatively with an eating disorder and will make it difficult for you to benefit from the programme. If you suffer from clinical depression, you may think it is impossible to change. You may have little energy to engage in treatment, and your poor concentration may make it difficult for you to understand and retain information. If you answer yes to any of these questions, you may be suffering from both an eating disorder and clinical depression:

- Did you have clinical depression before the onset of the eating disorder?
- Have your depressive symptoms (e.g., low mood, social withdrawal and suicidal thoughts and plans) recently got worse, but your eating-disorder features stayed the same?
- Have you lost interest in life or do you have recurrent thoughts on the uselessness of life?
- Are you crying all the time and have stopped looking after yourself?

If this is the case, talk to your therapist. If they decide you do have clinical depression, they will likely suggest that you take antidepressants. Opting for drugs rather than psychotherapy is best for two reasons: (1) psychotherapy takes a long time and it is essential that your eating disorder is treated now; (2) antidepressant drugs generally work well. Drugs specific for young people will be prescribed, as long as you and your parents agree.

Substance use disorder

Persistent substance misuse undermines your ability to make the most of treatment. If you have this problem, your therapist will refer you to a clinical centre specialising in substance use disorder treatment.

Competing commitments

School pressures or other commitments may have taken away from the time you could devote to the programme. Remember that CBT-E only works if you give priority to it. Carefully consider the pros and cons of shelving your other commitments for a while and considering the programme as a priority.

Coexisting psychological problems

Some psychological issues associated with the eating disorder (e.g., clinical perfectionism, core low self-esteem, marked interpersonal difficulties and mood intolerance—see Chapter 3) tend to maintain it and create an obstacle to the treatment. In this case, the broad form of CBT-E (see Chapter 5 and Part 3) may be better for you and recommended at this stage.

Dislike of CBT-E

If you have been treated with other forms of therapy (e.g., family therapy, psychodynamic psychotherapy or treatments based on the disease model), you might have difficulty adjusting to the CBT-E approach. If this is your problem, try to suspend your scepticism and simply accept that this is a science-based treatment with a good chance of helping you if you commit to it.

Reviewing your personal formulation

Taking stock is the ideal occasion to conduct a formal, detailed review of your personal formulation with your therapist. Together you will go over your monitoring records and the EPCL score summary sheet, looking at weekly changes. This joint review will highlight any emerging eating-disorder maintenance mechanisms, and any that you have already overcome. Your formulation can then be updated with this new information. If many changes need to be made to your formulation, it might be better to redraw it on a new sheet of paper.

If you are progressing, there will be no need to change track, but if it emerges that your mood intolerance, interpersonal issues, perfectionism and/or low self-esteem are getting in your way, it may be time to switch to broad CBT-E. This is an important decision because it will influence both the form and content of your treatment going forward. As such, you and your therapist will discuss the risks and benefits in depth before you make the decision together.

Planning Step Two

Step Two addresses the key maintenance mechanisms of your eating disorder while you continue to implement the strategies and procedures introduced in Step One. There are seven key maintenance mechanism components in eating disorders. As we discussed in Chapter 3, each of these psychological and behavioural features feed into the eating disorder, making it difficult to get rid of:

- Low weight and undereating
- Excessive exercising
- Purging
- Overvaluation of shape and weight
- Overvaluation of control over eating
- Dietary restraint
- Changes in eating triggered by moods or events

These will vary from individual to individual, but you will discuss all of them with your therapist to see which apply to you. After reviewing how and to what extent these seven maintenance mechanisms apply to you, you will decide with your therapist the order in which to tackle them. CBT-E has a specific module for breaking each of the above maintenance chains. These are described in the following chapters.

If you are low weight, or have lost a lot of weight and have starvation symptoms (see Chapter 3), it is recommended that you start with the Low Weight and Undereating module. This is because of the terrible consequences that your low weight and undereating are having on your physical health and psychosocial functioning. As we have already seen, they are also powerful processes maintaining your eating disorder. Suppose you are still using other extreme weight-control behaviours like excessive exercising, vomiting or misusing laxatives or diuretics. In that case, the Low Weight and Undereating module should be combined from the beginning with the Excessive Exercising and/or Purging modules as they are also obstacles to weight regain and can cause severe physical complications.

Then, after you have regained some weight, if you feel intense concerns about your shape and weight, the next step will be to implement the Body Image module. If you tend to use strict dietary rules, you will also start the Dietary Restraint module around this time. The Dietary Restraint module also includes specific strategies designed to tackle the overvaluation of eating control.

The Events, Moods and Eating module should be used only if events and associated mood changes are getting in the way of your recovery. Finally, the Setbacks and Mindsets module is introduced towards the end of Step Two. Figure 15.1 shows the order in which the CBT-E Modules are usually introduced in low-weight people with eating disorders.

If you are not low weight, it is advisable to start with the Body Image module. Body image is likely your most powerful maintenance mechanism, and it will require considerable time and effort to overcome. Once you are getting to grips with your body image concerns, you and your therapist will decide whether to move on to tackling your dietary restraint or mood issues. Generally speaking, the Dietary Restraint module is introduced a week or two after you have begun to work on body image. However, if you experience frequent episodes of binge eating triggered by events or moods, it is best to start the Events, Moods and Eating module first. Otherwise, you will start tackling events and moods a week or two after beginning to deal with dietary restraint.

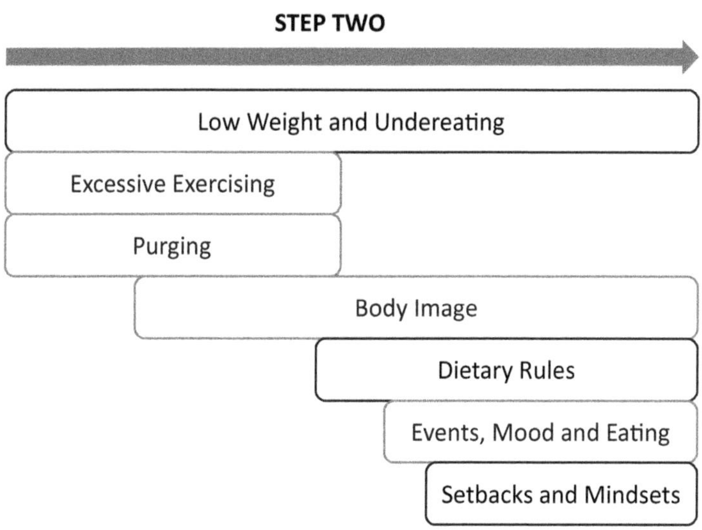

Figure 15.1 The order in which the CBT-E modules are usually introduced in people with an eating disorder and low weight. You will be offered the modules that apply to you.

As suggested for underweight people, if you adopt extreme weight-control behaviours (e.g., excessive exercising, vomiting, misusing laxatives), these should be addressed at the beginning of Step Two. Finally, the Setbacks and Mindsets module is introduced towards the end of Step Two.

In summary

At the end of Step One, after four weeks, in one or two sessions you and your therapist will jointly assess the progress you have made so far and decide which problems to address in Step Two. This review is repeated every four weeks during Step Two if you are restoring weight. These review sessions are dedicated to:

- Reviewing your progress
- Identifying your barriers to change
- Updating your personal formulation
- Deciding whether to switch to broad CBT-E
- Planning which and in which order to tackle the seven key eating-disorder maintenance mechanisms

• Take-home message

Don't take your foot off the accelerator! In Step Two, as in Step One, you should make your treatment a priority and maintain your momentum towards change.

16

Low Weight and Undereating module

The Low Weight and Undereating module will be your first if you are underweight or have lost a lot of weight and have starvation symptoms. This is a turning point in your treatment, and in your life. It is essential that you make the decision to restore your weight before beginning this module.

Information about weight restoration

Many concerns people have about weight regain are ill-founded. What you have picked up from friends or social media may be just plain wrong. It is important that you really understand what is involved in regaining weight. Knowing what to expect may help you feel in control during the process. The main points you should know are described next.

The psychology of weight regain

When you start the process of weight regain, you should be aware of the following points:

- Weight restoration is a long and demanding journey. You need to dedicate the same level of commitment that you were using to control your shape, weight and eating to the weight restoration process.
- Weight regain is associated with several short-term benefits, but the full benefits will only be appreciated once weight is fully restored and maintained for some years. Although partial weight restoration is also a considerable effort, it will not allow you to experience the full benefits of weight normalisation.
- Regaining weight is challenging, but it is worth it. When you reach a normal weight, you will feel free from the eating-disorder mindset and be ready to start a new life.

DOI: 10.4324/9781003342489-18

How much weight do I have to put on to be healthy?

The aim of the programme, and this module in particular, is for you to reach what call a "low healthy weight." Your healthy weight is determined by your genes and your biology. Any attempt to change it triggers a powerful biological response. Your body always wants to get back to the weight you were before. Your eating disorder challenges the process of maintaining a normal biological weight, and even if you do manage to get to a weight below your natural weight, you will pay a very high price. Losing a lot of weight causes you to develop starvation symptoms—these are the body's way of telling you to put the weight back on. Your preoccupation with food develops because your body knows it needs food to survive, and therefore that is the only thing you should be concerned with. However, if you have an eating disorder, you will likely interpret this biological drive to eat as a signal that you are somehow failing in your attempt to control your weight and shape. Instead of prompting you to eat, the increased hunger you feel as a result of malnourishment may cause you to increase your efforts to restrict your diet, fuelling the eating disorder cycle.

In order to make your starvation symptoms disappear, and therefore give you the chance to regain control of your eating, you will need to restore your weight to the low end of the healthy weight range. A low healthy weight fulfils the following four conditions:

1. It can be maintained without extreme weight-control behaviours.
2. It is not associated with starvation symptoms.
3. It is compatible with physical health and development.
4. It permits a social life.

In other words, a low healthy weight is a weight that no longer contributes to the maintenance of your eating disorder, and does not cause physical or psychosocial harm. According to the CBT-E, a low healthy weight needs to be identified with the help of your therapist once you reach the "minimum weight threshold," generally a BMI of 19.0 or the corresponding BMI-for-age percentile (see Chapter 10).

How will I go about it?

You will aim to establish a daily energy surplus sufficient to regain weight at a reasonable rate. You should expect to gain about 0.5 kilograms (1 lb) a week. The sooner you begin weight regain, the faster you will reach your goal weight range.

The amount of energy surplus involved in weight restoration is high. To regain weight at an average rate of 0.5 kilogram per week, you will need to consume, on average, an extra 500 kilocalories of energy each day (i.e., an extra 3,500 kilocalories per week) over and above what you needed to maintain a stable weight. However, if you increase your level of physical activity, you will need to increase your energy intake to match.

You may be afraid that your weight will shoot up beyond your control, but this will not happen. Gaining weight requires a lot of effort and weeks of constant work. It will not get out of hand. When you realise how difficult it is to regain weight, your fear of gaining weight uncontrollably will gradually disappear.

That being said, your rate of weight regain may be higher than 0.5 kilograms per week in the first week or two. This will be due to rehydration (i.e., water retention). Just as when you first start to diet, the water weight is the first thing to go, when you start to regain weight, it is the first thing you put back on. Remember that if you are undereating, you are probably dehydrated.

Strategies for regaining weight

Overcoming undereating and weight regain is difficult, but it is a necessary step on the road to recovery. You need to eliminate starvation symptoms and shatter the eating-disorder mindset. Most people with eating disorders believe that they will lose control and gain weight unpredictably if they eat certain foods or specific amounts of food. This belief causes anxiety and likely makes you undereat or adopt other extreme weight-control behaviours to make yourself feel better about yourself. However, as we have seen, these behaviours in turn maintain and intensify your preoccupation with eating. CBT-E helps you to address these preoccupations using the following strategies, all of which require your active involvement:

- Measuring and interpreting your weight
- Planning meals and snacks for regaining weight
- Real-time self-monitoring of eating
- Using cognitive behavioural strategies to overcome difficulties during meals
- Managing time after meals

Measuring and interpreting your weight

By Step Two, if your body weight is low, you will have had plenty of practice at weekly weighing and the correct way to interpret your weight. In Step Two, you should be using your weight chart to check that you are regaining weight at the reasonable rate of 0.5 kilograms per week. To help

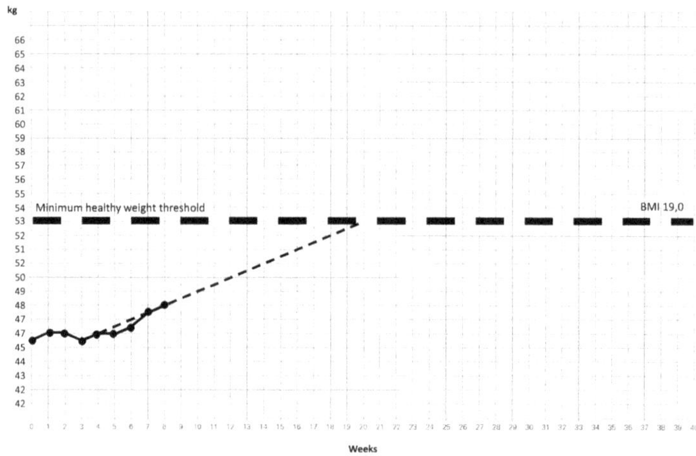

Figure 16.1 An example of a weight chart with weight regain trajectory drawn in

you correctly interpret weight regain, your therapist will draw a diagonal line on your weight chart from your latest weight up to the target minimum threshold weight (that corresponding to a BMI of 19.0 or a corresponding BMI-for-age percentile). This line should have a slope corresponding to an average rate of weight gain of 0.5 kilograms per week. A representative weight chart is shown in Figure 16.1. The slope of the diagonal line represents the expected rate of weight regain. Is your weight gain above or below this line?

As in Step One, you should interpret changes in your weight not relying on weekly readings but instead using the weight over the last four weeks. Is your rate of weight regain in line with the goal of about 0.5 kilograms a week? Weighing and interpreting your weight weekly will allow you to experience weight regain as a predictable and controlled process. It will help you dispel the belief that eating certain foods or amounts of foods will produce uncontrolled weight gain. Rather than losing control, you will see that you are gaining it.

Planning meals and snacks

CBT-E involves you actively planning the eating changes you need to make to regain weight. This will require you consuming more energy in the form of food and drink. You will already have a regular eating schedule, and now that you know when to eat, we will focus on what and how much. Together with your therapist or a CBT-E dietician, you will draw up a flexible meal plan. The foods you plan to eat will be acceptable to you and will produce the necessary initial daily energy surplus of 500 kcal.

In our clinic, we make use of a set of example daily menus as a guide, each containing three meals (i.e., breakfast, lunch and dinner) and two snacks, and all the food groups. Each menu has a mean daily calorie content calculated based on a weekly average: Menu A has about 1,500 kilocalories per day, Menu B has about 2,000 kilocalories per day, Menu C has about 2,500 kilocalories per day and Menu D has about 3,000 kilocalories per day. The idea is that you start with Menu A, then, if your weight is increasing by less than 0.5 kilograms per week, you switch to the next menu (e.g., Menu B, then Menu C and so on).

However, the idea is not to fixate on calorie counting. You will be aiming for a rough weekly average, not a fixed amount each day. You and your therapist (or CBT-E dietician) will draw up a weekly meal plan with all the five food groups (i.e., fruit and vegetables, starchy food, dairy, protein, fat), which you will be encouraged to include in your meals. You will be free to choose what type of food to eat within the food group. For example, it does not matter whether you get your proteins from fish or meat, as long as you get your proteins. As far as portions are concerned, these will be based on those normally consumed by people without an eating disorder. In this phase of treatment, it is best that you have your meals together with a parent or other adult family member (maybe a grandparent). It is also better during the early stages of weight regain to eat your main meals at home rather than at school or work, if possible. Mid-morning and mid-afternoon snacks can and should, however, be consumed where you are at those times.

Every week, you will interpret your emerging weight trend over the previous four weeks, as in Step One. If you have eaten your planned meals and snacks, and your weight is increasing by less than 0.5 kg per week, you will decide with your therapist to raise your daily calorie intake by 500 kcal per day. You will plan together the changes required to maintain the agreed rate of weight regain of 0.5 kilograms per week. During the week, you will write in advance (the day before) when, what and where to eat at the top of your monitoring record (using the first three columns) and draw a line at the end of the daily plan. Take a look at "Today's Plan" drawn up by Amanda and her therapist, which is shown in Figure 16.2.

Implementing this procedure provides you with an eating structure and allows you to address some dietary rules (e.g., not eating certain food groups). It also permits you to feel in control during the process of weight regain as you can predict the increase in your weight (e.g., "If I follow Menu B, my body weight will increase by about 0.5 kg in a week") and dispel the belief that eating certain foods or amounts of foods will produce uncontrolled weight gain.

Day Thursday **Date** 10th October

Time	Food and drinks consumed	Place	*	V/L/E	Context and comments
	Today's plan				
7:00	I cup of whole milk I tablespoon of sugar I muffin I orange juice	Kitchen			
10:30	I apple	School			
13:30	I plate of pasta with tomato and I spoon of parmesan I portion of chicken I serving of zucchini I spoon of olive oil	Kitchen			
16:30	I ice-cream	Bar			
20:00	I portion of salmon 2 slices of wholemeal bread I serving of salad I spoon of olive oil I orange	Kitchen			
7:00	I cup of yogurt I tablespoon of sugar I muffin I orange juice	Kitchen			As I planned. I feel fine. I skipped the apple. Nobody else is eating a snack and they are all thinner than me. If I ate the apple, I would feel guilty because the other guys are not eating
13:30	I plate of spaghetti with tomato and parmesan I portion of chicken I serving of zucchini I spoon of olive oil	Kitchen			Quiet lunch, although I'm a little concerned that by eating spaghetti I will get fat
16:30	I apple	Kitchen			I'm eating an apple instead of the ice-cream. Ice-cream is fattening and I'm afraid of putting on weight too fast.
20:00	I portion of salmon 2 slices of wholemeal bread I serving of salad I spoon of olive oil I pear	Kitchen			There were no oranges left so I had a pear instead . No problem

Figure 16.2 An example of a monitoring record, filled in by Amanda during her weight regain phase

Self-monitoring eating in real time

It is important that you continue to keep your monitoring record on the table while eating and filling it in in real time. Stick to the procedure you learned in Step One (see Chapter 10).

Using cognitive behavioural strategies to handle difficulties during meals

Usually, your active involvement in interpreting weight regain (see above) and planning meals and snacks to regain weight will reduce your anxiety and concerns about eating and food. This procedure has been designed to help you to experience weight regain as a predictable and controlled process and to dispel your belief that eating certain types or amounts of food will produce uncontrolled weight gain. Eating a broad range of foods also helps you to understand that "a calorie is a calorie" and that there are no foods that cannot be part of a healthy diet.

However, it is important that you practise doing one or more of the following things if you get into difficulties at mealtimes:

- *Eat everything you planned to eat.* Stick to the plan and you will regain weight at an appropriate rate. Take control and you will feel in control.
- *Urge surfing.* At times you will be tempted to ignore what you agreed to do with your therapist. This would be a mistake. For a while, you will have to actively fight against these urges using techniques such as urge surfing (see Chapter 12), and do the opposite of what they are telling you to do.
- *Do not let feelings of hunger and fullness influence what you eat.* Remember that your hunger signals are distorted by your low weight and are therefore not a good guide on what, when and how much to eat.
- *Do not be influenced by recurrent thoughts about food and eating.* These are your eating disorder mindset talking. You cannot rely on them to tell you what, when or how much to eat.
- *Eat normally.* You may have got into the habit of eating very slowly, cutting food into small pieces or other abnormal food rituals. The tendency to eat in these strange ways is due to your eating disorder. Try to eat in the same way as others do. This will help you regain weight at an appropriate rate.
- *If you are having difficulties eating, record them (in real time) on your monitoring record.* This will let us come up with solutions to your problems.

Remember that the programme's purpose is to help you regain (and eventually maintain) a healthy weight in a predictable and controlled way.

Managing time after eating

After a meal you should do something to distract yourself from the urge to engage in compensatory behaviours. Before a meal, plan to read, watch TV, study, listen to music or surf the net afterwards—anything that will take your mind off vomiting or excessive exercising. If you are in the habit of vomiting after meals, avoid the bathrooms for an hour after eating. If you tend to exercise excessively, plan to put your feet up for at least an hour after eating. If the urge to vomit or exercise comes upon you, take deep, slow breaths and remember to apply your coping techniques (like you did with regular eating in Chapter 12).

Other strategies that can help you tackle weight regain

Wardrobe changes

During the process of regaining weight, the clothes you are wearing now may well become too small. Know that this will happen and don't panic when it does. In fact, you can prevent the problem arising in the first place by wearing loose-fitting clothes during the weight gain process or buying new "less small" clothing at regular intervals. This is a good idea because clothes that are too tight increase body awareness. This may intensify your concerns about your weight and body shape and make it more difficult to stay on track. It is, therefore, best to remind yourself of the following:

- Planning for your shape changes and buying new clothes before the old ones become tight is a way of staying in control.
- The positive things about increasing clothing size, namely shopping (who doesn't love shopping?), having a greater range of clothes and looking better in them.
- To fit into your current clothes, you would need to stay ill.

If your existing wardrobe is looking rather dull and dated, ask your friends or family to help you buy clothing that is more trendy and "you." Think about what you would advise a friend to wear. In fact, this could help your recovery process. Going shopping with a friend who does not have an eating disorder can improve your shape acceptance. It is also a way of working against your social withdrawal.

Don't keep your old clothes. You should burn your bridges by giving them away. Think of someone wanting to keep clothes from a period in their life during which they were severely ill, like suffering from cancer. Would they want to have a constant reminder of this period in their life, or is it truly time for a fresh start? What about you?

Dealing with feeling full

Feeling full is a problem frequently experienced during weight restoration. To prevent it from becoming a barrier to change for you, fill in the "Context and Comments" column of your monitoring record at the precise moment you experience the feeling of fullness. This real-time self-monitoring should help you understand why you are feeling this way. Then you will be able to analyse with your therapist which of these things are true for you (sometimes there may be more than one):

1. *Thinking you have eaten too much.* This is probably because you have a distorted view of how much food is an appropriate amount. Refer back to

your meal plan and your dietary recommendations and look at how much other people around you are eating.

2. *Feeling there is too much food in your stomach*. This is a physical experience that everybody has every day. It does not mean you have eaten too much or put on weight. Remember that low weight and undereating slow your digestion, increasing the intensity of feeling full.
3. *Clothing feeling abnormally tight*. Outgrowing your clothes is inevitable during weight regain. It is the consequence of the natural changes in shape that you are aiming for. This feeling does not mean that you have overeaten or gotten fat, and in any case it will pass. Make sure that you are not wearing clothes that are too small that need to be replaced (see "Wardrobe Changes," above).
4. *Feeling fat*. Feeling full is not the same as feeling fat (or being fat). If this is a problem for you, and is getting in the way of your recovery, it might be a good idea to start the Body Image module (Chapter 19). Indeed, if you equate feeling full with feeling fat, if you don't do something about it, this may increase your concerns about shape, weight and eating control, triggering dietary restriction or other extreme weight-control behaviours.

After you and your therapist have identified the nature of your feelings of fullness, you will be encouraged to try one or more of the following strategies:

- *Wear looser clothes*. Tight clothes may make you feel full, even if you have only eaten a little. Wear something that doesn't press on your stomach.
- *Don't trust the feeling of fullness*. Undereating and low weight slow digestion, which can intensify the normal feeling of fullness you get after a meal. Do not let your fullness or hunger dictate how much you eat, as one or both sensations are likely to be disrupted by the eating disorder. Once you are eating regularly (three meals plus two snacks a day) and regaining weight, your digestion will return to normal. This may take a few months, but it is only temporary.
- *Remember it will pass*. Acknowledge to yourself that feeling full is temporary and natural. Feeling full is a physical experience that everybody has every day. It is caused by food in the stomach, not fat. It does not mean you have eaten too much or put on weight.
- *Deal with it*. Remember that *feeling* full or fat is not the same *being* fat. The Body Image module has some excellent strategies that will help you cope with this feeling.

Dealing with belly shape

It is common for your stomach to stick out a little when you start to regain weight. This is because, in the initial stages of weight restoration, fat is deposited in the abdominal area. Don't panic, and don't start body checking.

Behaviours like looking down at your belly when sitting or pinching it after eating will only intensify your concerns about shape and weight. Be aware that your stomach may appear to stick out if you wear certain clothes, reintroduce fibre to your diet or drink a lot of carbonated drinks. Use the following tips to help you get over this potential stumbling block:

- *Wear clothes that are not tight around the belly.*
- *Reduce your intake of fizzy drinks.*
- *Remember that these feelings and perceptions are exaggerated because you have an eating disorder and are underweight.*
- *Don't check the shape of your stomach.* Don't look down at it while you are eating, and don't look in the mirror afterwards.
- *If you do happen look at your stomach from above*, try to look down at other people's bellies while they are sitting down. To do this you will need to look over their shoulder. This should help you understand that nobody is looking at your stomach from this perspective—that would be weird!
- *See if you notice any differences in the size of other people's bellies after they have eaten.* If you don't see significant differences—you won't—this test can help you see that people do not notice or look for changes in the size of other people's bellies after eating. Once again, that would be weird.

Dealing with feeling bloated

The feeling of being bloated is a common physical sensation, especially in women in the premenstrual phase. It is due to an increase in water retention. This is also why it occurs in people with eating disorders when they restore their water weight after a long period of dehydration, start regular eating and stop self-induced vomiting and/or taking laxatives and diuretics. The sensation may be particularly bothersome in the early stages of weight restoration, especially if your legs are affected.

However, bear in mind that feeling bloated does not mean that you have eaten too much. Feeling bloated, like feeling full, is not the same as being fat. Be aware that if you fall into this way of thinking, it can maintain the eating disorder. Do not let it intensify your concerns about eating, shape and weight, and do not be tempted to increase dietary restraint or take water pills.

Also, it may be that your cycle is starting up again, and what you are experiencing is premenstrual fluid retention. Try to tolerate this state for a few days, and remember that it is water weight, not fat. It is only a temporary increase.

Similarly, if your legs swell a bit once you start eating properly, try to have a little patience, as it usually disappears within a few days. Your body requires a little time to get used to this new, healthier physical state. Keeping your legs raised may make the swelling go down. If they are very swollen, though, you should talk to your doctor, who may be able to prescribe you specific drugs to treat this condition.

If you are feeling bloated but are not actually swelling up, this is probably because you are not used to living with a normally hydrated body. Keep calm, and within a few days, your body will get used to having enough water.

Whatever the case, do not use diuretics, laxatives, self-induced vomiting or dietary restriction in response to feeling bloated. These strategies only temporarily reduce the sensation of being bloated. Meanwhile, they create a state of dehydration that will make you feel even more bloated as soon as you rehydrate. Resist the urge! It is a temporary hurdle that you will have to get over to get well.

FAQs on weight restoration

What about my dietary rules?

If you have been following extreme dietary rules that exclude food groups, your therapist or CBT-E dietician will want to talk to you about this. You will be given nutritional education and advice based on your country's food and nutrition guidelines, with suggestions for meals and snacks. The goal is to devise a flexible plan involving the consumption of foods that are acceptable to you and will produce the necessary initial daily energy surplus of 500 kilocalories. Remember that the foods you have been avoiding will not actually hurt you, and you have decided to eat healthily to regain weight. This will necessarily involve eating all the food groups.

What if I'm not putting on weight?

If you are already sticking to your plan and your weight has remained stable across the last four weeks, know that this is normal. Remember that starvation symptoms slow your metabolism, and as you regain weight, your resting energy expenditure goes up. If this is slowing your progress, increasing your calorie intake to keep pace will be necessary, switching to the next menu (e.g., from Menu B to Menu C and so on). To help you, your therapist may also provide a list of foods (or food combinations) that contain 500 kilocalories of energy. You can then choose to supplement your usual diet with items from the list to create an energy surplus of 500 kilocalories each day. If you find that this is difficult or ineffective, you and your therapist might consider whether to boost your energy intake by using energy drinks. These are a quick and easy way to get your extra calories, as they usually contain about 250 kilocalories per carton or bottle. So, if you drink two of these a day, your weight should go up by about 0.5 kilograms per week. Used wisely, these drinks have several advantages. First, they provide the energy surplus needed without requiring overeating. Second, they can be easily eliminated once you reach your target BMI range, so you won't need to cut back on eating. Third, they couldn't be any simpler to use. However, energy drinks can make you feel full, so it's better to drink them after eating than before. For example, you could try drinking one after breakfast and one after your mid-afternoon snack.

What if I'm a vegetarian or vegan?

If you are a vegetarian or vegan, your therapist will ask you about your reasons for being so, as vegetarian and vegan diets are sometimes a feature of an eating disorder. If you started your vegetarian or vegan diets as a means of controlling eating, you should address these dietary rules using standard CBT-E procedures (see the Dietary Restraint module). As with any other form of food avoidance, they are a powerful maintenance mechanism of your eating disorder.

If, on the other hand, you don't eat meat or animal products for religious or ethical reasons, you should carefully assess with your therapist the pros and cons of suspending vegetarianism or veganism for a few months. This will be giving yourself a better chance of overcoming your eating disorder. If you are not prepared to accept this temporary suspension, a CBT-E dietician will be able to help you devise a healthy and flexible vegetarian or vegan diet.

Restoring weight requires a continuous effort for many months. You will often be tempted to give up before you reach your goal weight range. As this is highly inadvisable, below is a list of common problems and how to address them.

Common difficulties with weight restoration

Motivation issues

It is normal for your motivation to wax and wane somewhat, but to nip any problems in the bud, you will need to explore these with your therapist on a weekly basis. Think about any changes in motivation you have noticed over the week and what may have influenced these changes.

You must also go over again with your therapist your reasons for wanting to restore weight. It may be useful to write these reasons on a sheet of paper to keep on the table while you are eating. Remember the harm your eating disorder causes to your life, remind yourself of your short- and medium-term goals and identify what you find more difficult than your peers.

Being in two minds about change is understandable, but now you have a real possibility of overcoming your eating disorder. You have at least five opportunities to choose to get better (or not) each day before each of your planned meals and snacks, and it is these choices that will determine your progress.

Weight gain can be compared to a long and difficult journey that will lead you to a healthy place where you can live a happy life full of opportunities. Imagine you are in canoe, paddling downstream. You pass some other people who tell you that you are going the wrong way—there is a fabulous, must-see beauty spot in the other direction, while the way you are going there is only a polluted stretch of water surrounded by factories. To get to the beauty spot you will have to turn your canoe round and row against the current. What do you do?

You are in a similar position with your eating disorder. You trust that your therapist is right when they tell you that recovering from your eating disorder will be a wonderful thing, but you are finding it hard work to stop dieting and increase your energy intake—to row against the current. You know that you will have to do it for a long time to reach your destination—the goal of low and healthy weight. However, if you stop rowing, you will be dragged back by the current and will have even further to go tomorrow. You will have put in a lot of effort, but your destination will be out of reach. Remember that you will only feel the benefits of weight restoration when you reach a low healthy weight. The weight regain process is hard, but the result will be worth the effort. What are you going to do?

Forgetting your reasons for regaining weight

In some people, the eating-disorder mindset reasserts itself as soon as they have left the therapist's office. This may cause them to forget why they want to restore their weight mere minutes after the end of the session. If you have this problem, you should keep a list of your reasons for change close to hand and read through it regularly, particularly when you sit down to eat and get up in the morning, as well as in "emergency" situations.

The changes you are making are too small

You may feel the urge to put the brakes on and take fairy steps as opposed to regular strides, especially when it comes to eating. This is a common occurrence, but put yourself in the canoe again—how are you ever going to get there if you use half an oar?

Do your best to stick to your eating plan. If you eat less than you planned, you will never put the weight on and never get well. All you will be doing is rowing to stay in the same place. Be honest with your therapist, who will be able to help you explore your reasons for doing so. You may be overestimating the energy content of certain foods, which may prompt you to eat too little. You may feel that making small changes is "safer," that there is less risk of you overdoing it and putting on too much weight. This is especially likely if you are eating foods you are unused to eating, or those whose calorie content is difficult to assess. In reality, though, it is not eating enough that is "unsafe," because it will stop you overcoming your eating disorder. Your fear of overeating is unjustified. Your eating plan has been specifically designed to provide a controlled rate of weight regain. Furthermore, it usually takes just as much effort to make large changes as it does to make smaller ones.

You are concerned about getting fat

You need to ask yourself whether this is actually the case. FYI: it is not. Even in the worst-case scenario, you will change from **emaciated** to slim. Nonetheless, the difficulty you may have in accepting your new shape is understandable. If you feel that parts of your body are getting unacceptably "fat," talk to your therapist about it. They will help you understand, reinterpret and override this feeling. This will likely involve working on your body image as you work on healthy eating (see the Body Image module in Chapter 19), enabling you to more easily accept weight regain.

> JARGON BUSTER
>
> **emaciated** (adjective): abnormally thin or weak

You are worried about eating unhealthily

If you develop this belief, talk to your therapist or dietician about it. In your emaciated state it is your low weight, rather than energy-rich food, that is dangerous. The normal rules of healthy eating do not apply when you are underweight. General dietary guidelines are not designed for people with an eating disorder, who will only recover by eating energy-rich foods. Once you have reached your goal weight range, you will be free to limit your consumption of such foods if you wish, provided that you avoid high levels of dietary restraint and eat enough to maintain your weight. Now is not the time to worry about such things.

You think you have gained enough weight (but are still underweight)

When you start approaching your target weight range, you may feel you can stop rowing. Although you should praise yourself for your efforts so far, the battle is not yet won. If you stop now, you will never get to your destination and be able to enjoy all the benefits of weight restoration. Though you have put on some weight, and will therefore be less unhealthy than when you started the journey, this is no place to stop. Maintaining an unhealthily low body weight will not enable you to overcome your eating-disorder mindset permanently. This will leave you at significant risk of relapse. Moreover, should you lose any weight due to illness, etc., you will be thrust straight back into the "danger zone" before you know it.

Going from weight restoration to weight maintenance

When you reach the minimal BMI threshold (a BMI of 19.0), you will begin to discuss the topic of weight maintenance with your therapist. At this point, you should collaboratively identify with your therapist your healthy weight-maintenance range. This will meet the four conditions described at the beginning of this chapter, specifically:

1. It can be maintained without extreme weight-control behaviours.
2. It is not associated with starvation symptoms.
3. It is compatible with physical health and development.
4. It permits a social life.

An important piece of information to remember is that your weight will never be fixed point—it normally fluctuates by 2–3 kg due to natural variations in the body's water content. For this reason, weight maintenance will involve you learning to maintain a stable weight with a range of approximately 3 kilograms above the minimum low healthy weight. You will probably devote at least 6–8 weeks to reaching this goal.

The psychology of weight maintenance

In comparison to weight restoration, maintenance is relatively simple. If you gain weight at the appropriate rate, it is simply a matter of slightly reducing the amount of food you are eating without undereating. This must be done with caution, however, as there is a risk that you could lose weight if you go overboard. If you have been using daily energy drinks to boost your weight regain, you should eliminate one when you are close to your identified minimum healthy weight threshold and the second when you reach it.

The goal is for you to maintain a weight within a range of about 3 kilograms (see Federica's example in Figure 16.3), and to do so, you need to learn how to balance your activity levels and energy intake. You will be surprised at how much you can eat without gaining weight. It is important to note that at this stage, patients and therapists have very different concerns. While your therapist may be focused on helping you maintain a healthy weight, you may be afraid that your weight will continue to rise. You may therefore be tempted to take preventative action, potentially cutting down too far. However, it is important to prevent any attempt to lose weight; otherwise, you will fall into

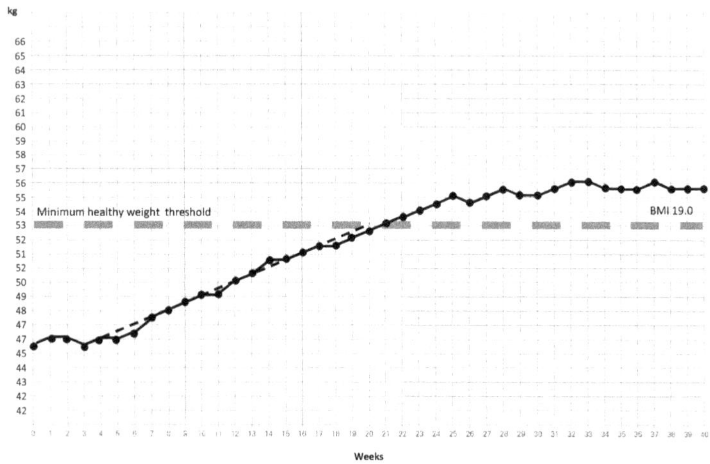

Figure 16.3 An example weight chart filled in by Federica, who was underweight when she started the programme, but has now completed both the weight regain and the weight maintenance phase

weight-loss pitfall, potentially reactivating your eating-disorder mindset. It would be a bit like rowing downstream while facing upstream. Trust that your meal plans will get you where you need to be, just as they did before. If your weight doesn't remain stable, they can always be adjusted. The trick is to stay focused, and stay on track.

It is also vital during the weight-maintenance phase that you and your therapist continue to address your **residual** eating-disorder features. You should also make an effort to accept and take pleasure in your new appearance and adjust to emerging aspects of your unique personality, which may be very different from what you once thought it was.

> JARGON BUSTER
>
> **residual** (adjective): remaining, leftover

Melanie's story

I was a mess in my early teens. My parents divorced when I was 8 years old and me and my twin brother ended up living with my da while my ma went off and made a new happy family. I was pretty miserable and had no friends. I hated school and was teased all the time for being fat and stupid. I did a lot of comfort eating to make me feel better and by the end of middle school I weighed 70 kg. I didn't want to be that fat when I started high school, so I went to see a nutritionist. I did what they told me and got my weight down to 54 kg in six months. I didn't stop there, though, and got down to 40 kg. I think it was because being able to control my weight made me feel better about myself. I didn't think I had a problem, but my da made me go to a specialist eating-disorder centre. They gave me antidepressants and a diet plan, which I didn't stick to. My da made the meals up for me before he went to work, but I'd just eat a few vegetables, sling the rest in the bin, and tell him I'd eaten the lot. I'd cover the scraps up with other rubbish so he never found out. My brother was always out with his pals, so he didn't know either. One day though my da came home and found me collapsed on my bedroom floor, and the ambulance came and took me off to the hospital. They kept me in there for a month, until I put on a couple of kilos, but when I got out I went back to my old ways. I wanted to restore some weight because I was scared of dying, but I could only eat like a bird. I was 19, out of work and with no life. I started feeling dizzy again, so I went down the doctor's. She sent me to a CBT-E, which was brilliant. I got through Step One with no bother, but then things went wrong. I understood the stuff about maintenance mechanisms and that things needed to change, but I was basically waiting for the change to happen to me, not through me. When I started Step Two, I stuck to my meal plan, but didn't put on any weight because I just couldn't eat everything on my plate. My therapist asked me about this and I said that I felt so full after a few mouthfuls that I had to stop eating. She explained that feeling full was actually caused by my low weight and did not actually mean that I was full. She told me that when I put on weight my hunger signalling would get back to normal, and encouraged me to try to make normal portions and eat everything on my plate. Her advice on portion sizes was really helpful because before I'd been used to eating tiny amounts on my own, so it was good to know how much normal people eat. My da started coming home from work at lunch so he could eat three meals a day with me, which helped a lot. I wasn't stuck in the house on my own all day so I felt less lonely, too. Chatting with my da at mealtimes helped me to ignore my full feeling, and I started putting on weight and feeling better in myself and about myself.

In summary

The Low Weight and Undereating module is indicated if you have a low weight. The module has two main goals:

1. Weight restoration above the minimum low healthy weight. To achieve this goal, you need to consume, on average, an extra 500 kilocalories of energy each day over and above what you need to maintain a stable weight.

Followed by:

2. Weight maintenance within a range of approximately 3 kilograms above the minimum low healthy weight.

To help you feel in control during the weight regain, you will use the following strategies:

- Measuring and interpreting your weight
- Planning meals and snacks for regaining weight
- Real-time self-monitoring of eating
- Using cognitive behavioural strategies to overcome difficulties during meals
- Managing time after meals

• Take-home message

Regaining weight is challenging, but it is worth it. With weight normalisation, you will feel free from the eating-disorder mindset and be ready to start a new, better life.

Excessive Exercising module

The Excessive Exercising module should be implemented at the start of Step Two if you are still excessing excessively. It can be done at the same time as the Low Weight and Undereating module if you also have a low weight. As with the other procedures of CBT-E, it is essential that you make the decision to tackle excessive exercising before beginning this module.

Do I exercise excessively?

It will likely be obvious to your parents and therapist that you exercise excessively. You will probably do things like refusing to take the elevator or sit down in the waiting room or at home, which are dead giveaways. However, it may be more difficult for you to admit that you have this problem. The most common reason for this is that excessive exercising gets to be a habit. You may also consider your exercise to be healthy and indispensable for controlling your weight and body shape. So, it is important that you look for clues that you may be exercising excessively. Ask yourself the following questions:

- Does your exercise interfere with important activities like school or socialising?
- Do you exercise in strange places or at inappropriate times?
- Do you feel that you must exercise, even if it hurts?
- Does not exercising make you feel guilty?

If you answer yes to any one of these questions, it is likely that your exercising has gotten out of control. So that you and your therapist can understand the extent of the problem, they will suggest that you monitor your exercising habits using your monitoring record. You should record every time you exercise (including not sitting still) with a letter "E" in the "V/L/E" column, and then the type of exercise you did, how long you did it for and why you did it. Whether it was to control your weight and shape and/or to modulate mood, you should your record your reasons in the "Context and Comments" column.

DOI: 10.4324/9781003342489-19

Weighing up the pros and cons of stopping excessive exercising

We discussed excessive exercising in Chapter 3, so look back over that section if you need to refresh your memory on its harmful effects. From your therapist's perspective, you need to stop exercising excessively for two main reasons:

1. It causes significant damage to your body, mental health and social functioning.
2. It is a powerful eating-disorder maintenance mechanism.

As with the other features of your eating disorder that CBT-E is designed to help you tackle, it must be you who decides to interrupt your excessive exercising. Your parents and therapist may want you to stop, but only you can make the change. As you probably don't see your exercising as a problem, but rather as a positive way of controlling shape and weight or modulating mood, this is often a difficult task. However, it is an important decision, and if you are low weight, it should be made when you decide to tackle weight restoration, for obvious reasons.

Indeed, to help you make this decision, you will use a similar strategy to that you used to decide to tackle weight regain in Step One (see Chapter 13)—creating with your therapist a pros-and-cons-of-change table. As part of this process, it is crucial that you tell your therapist the positives that you feel your exercising brings to your life, and any doubts you may have about stopping. You can then fill in the left-hand column, listing all the cons of stopping. Consider whether exercising provides you with benefits that you would be afraid of losing. If you have a fear of losing control over your weight if you interrupt your exercising, don't worry. Adopting a healthy lifestyle with a balanced diet and moderate physical activity is the best way to control your weight in the long term.

Next, think about the advantages of changing in detail. Reflect on the short- and long-term effects of excessive exercising on your health, psychology, relationships and school/work or sports performance. Remember that change will be necessary if you are ever going to free yourself from the adverse effects of this type of exercise and break the chains of your eating disorder. Now you can fill in the right-hand column of your table with all your reasons for change. Repeat the procedure for six months to a year in the future, and then take your tables home to think about and update if necessary. By the next session, you should have made the decision that you would like to try and stop excessive exercising, which you can write down at the bottom of the sheet. Remember that if you decide not to do so, this programme cannot continue.

Strategies and procedures for tackling excessive exercising

When you have decided you do want to tackle your excessive exercising, you should agree with your therapist on which procedures to use. The main procedures adopted by CBT-E to address excessive exercising are the following:

- *Self-monitoring exercise in real time.* Write the events, thoughts and emotions that precede the start of exercising in real time in the "Context and Comments" column of your monitoring record. If you do this before you start exercising, you will become aware of what you are doing, thinking and feeling at the precise time that the urge to exercise strikes, making it easier for you to resist doing it.
- *Do healthy exercising.* It is essential that you break any link between eating and exercising, which means stopping any form of compensatory exercising (either before or after eating) cold turkey. However, if your doctor gives you the go-ahead, you should replace excessive exercising with healthy social exercise. This is because being "in good shape," both physically and mentally, puts you in the best position for overcoming excessive exercising. Try exercising in less extreme ways and doing so with friends. Social exercising is a valuable way to escape isolation (which, as you know, maintains eating disorders), so suggest to your friends that you meet up for tennis, dance lessons or yoga classes.
- *Tackling the urge to exercise.* As with tackling the urge to binge in Step One, make a list of "things to say and things to do," as described in Chapter 12. These should help you ride out the urge to exercise (urge surfing). To distract yourself, do something that will make exercising less likely, like watching a movie. The best activities for this purpose are those you can do with your friends.
- *Stopping competitive sports.* If you are underweight and practice a competitive sport, your therapist will likely ask you to put your training on hold. They will probably talk to your coach about encouraging you to temporarily suspend both practice and competitions. Indeed, an intense exercise regime, especially in high-level competitive sports, can be a powerful eating-disorder maintenance mechanism, as well as dangerous for health. In fact, the research indicates that rest and achieving a healthy weight are necessary to improve sports performance.
- *Managing events and associated mood changes that trigger exercising.* You may be using excessive exercising to make you feel better. This is a dysfunctional coping strategy, and you need to find healthier ways of dealing with your feelings—see the specific strategies described in the Events, Moods and Eating module.

- *Asking for help.* If the preceding procedures are not successful in helping you deal with the urge to exercise, you may need to recruit outside assistance. Your therapist may consider, with your consent, involving your parents or a trusted person to help you to at least limit your exercising using the same procedures described.

As with any other change, your anxiety and concern about shape and weight might go up in the first few days of tackling excessive exercising. But, when you start to get control, they will gradually fade, and you will start to feel the benefits of leading a healthy lifestyle.

Anthony's story

I started CBT-E when I was 24 years old. I wasn't very hopeful at first, because I'd already tried several different treatments and none of them had worked. I was unemployed at the time and living with my mother and brother. My father worked away from home and so was basically away all week.

The thing I liked about CBT-E was the fact that they wanted my input. The treatments I had tried before were a bit dehumanising, and I appreciated the opportunity to talk through my problems with my therapist and develop strategies for overcoming them together. My biggest problem was excessive exercising. Because I didn't have a job, I'd basically be cycling and doing push-ups all day. I was so focused on my physical appearance that I didn't think it was doing me any harm, but with my therapist's help I began to see that in order to improve my performance I would need to put on muscle mass, not burn it off. He suggested that I try to find other ways of getting satisfaction than the effort I was putting into exercising and the tiredness I felt afterwards.

I could see his point, so I shifted my focus to addressing weight regain and following the meal plan properly, but I had a constant niggling thought that I was putting on fat mass rather than lean mass. Secretly, I was convinced that I would never be able to achieve peak performance if I reached a BMI over 19. When I failed to start putting on weight, my therapist got this information out of me, and told me all the ways excessive exercising would be counterproductive in the long run. What really drove it home to me was him telling me that being underweight and exercising too much put me at a high risk of stress fractures and brittle bones—you can't ride a bike with a broken leg. That's mainly why I agreed it might be a good idea to start easing off on my exercising habits. The first step was to monitor what I was doing on a daily basis by writing it down on my monitoring record. I was also encouraged to think about the negative effects of my exercising, namely no job and no time for friends. It was also frustrating to me that my physical performance was getting worse, not better, and I was having to eating lots of fatty foods to balance out my energy expenditure, which worsened my fears about getting fat. After writing all this down in a pros and cons of change table, I could see that exercising so much was more detrimental to me than it was helpful, and so I really committed to cutting down, at least until I had put on weight. One massive milestone in this process was when I phoned up a few old university buddies and invited them to go bowling. Not only was it a lot of fun, but I was also able to channel my energies into a social sport that didn't stop me from reaching my weight restoration goals. Our team is now top of the league!

In summary

The Excessive Exercising module is designed to help you stop excessive exercising as a routine form of weight control. Excessive exercising needs to be addressed because it causes physical and mental damage and maintains the eating disorder.

If you exercise excessively, you probably:

- Do exercise that interferes with important activities
- Exercise in strange places or at inappropriate times
- Feel obliged to exercise, even if it hurts
- Feel guilty if you don't exercise

Once you have weighed up the pros and cons of stopping excessive exercising, you will make the decision to do so. The main procedures adopted by CBT-E to address excessive exercising are the following:

- Real-time self-monitoring of exercise
- Doing healthy physical activity
- Addressing the urge to exercise using "things to say and do"
- Putting competitive sports on hold
- Learning to deal with events and associated mood changes that trigger exercising

If all else fails, your parents or a trusted person can be recruited to help you limit your exercising.

• Take-home message

If you are offered this module, it is because the way you are exercising is harmful, not healthy. You need to stop it if you want to regain your physical, mental and social health.

18

Purging module

As we saw in Chapter 4, purging by self-induced vomiting and/or the misuse of laxatives (more rarely the misuse of diuretics, aka water pills) may be used as a "compensatory" or "non-compensatory" means of controlling weight. How we deal with it will depend on which purging behaviours you have. It may not even be addressed if you practice only compensatory purging. As you use this to "cancel out" specific episodes of perceived or actual overeating, it will tail off as you gain control over eating. If you practice non-compensatory purging as a routine weight-loss strategy, on the other hand, it may need special attention. This is because your purging is not so closely linked to the amount of food you eat and will not likely go away on its own once you are eating normally. As a general rule, this kind of purging needs to be addressed during treatment, especially as prolonged misuse of laxatives can lead to chronic constipation, which tends to increase concerns about eating and belly shape.

If you are still using non-compensatory purging to control your body weight at the start of Step Two, this is the time you will start the Purging module, along with the Low Weight and Undereating module if you also have a low weight. As with the other procedures of CBT-E, it is essential that you make the decision to tackle purging before beginning this module.

Monitoring purging

The first thing to do is to know your enemy. Let's get some things straight: self-induced vomiting and misuse of laxatives and diuretics do not make you lose weight in long-term. They are not an alternative to dieting. In order to get a handle on the situation, you will be asked to monitor your purging habits, recording all episodes with a letter "V" (vomiting) and/or "L" (laxatives) or "D" (diuretics) in the "V/L/E" column on your monitoring record as they happen. Alongside the type of purging you did, you should record the number of pills you took (if you took laxatives or diuretics), your reasons for doing it (to control weight and shape and/or to modulate mood) and whether it was compensatory or non-compensatory purging in the "Context and Comments" column.

DOI: 10.4324/9781003342489-20

Weighing up the pros and cons of stopping purging

Although at first you may think purging is an easy method of weight control, after a while, you will lose control over eating and end up binge-eating more frequently. This is why purging needs to be interrupted, in addition to two other reasons:

1. It has significant adverse effects on your physical health (see the sections "Physical Effects of Purging" in Chapter 4 for details).
2. It is a powerful eating-disorder maintenance mechanism (see the sections "Self-induced Vomiting" and "Laxative and Diuretics Misuse" in Chapter 3 for details).

> JARGON BUSTER
>
> **regurgitation** (noun): bringing swallowed food back up into the mouth

If you engage in purging behaviour that requires attention, such as non-compensatory purging (including spitting, with or without **regurgitation**), you will be helped by your therapist to weigh up your reasons for and against stopping. As with all CBT-E procedures, it is crucial that it is you who makes the decision to stop. To this end you should create with your therapist a pros-and-cons-of-change table, using a similar strategy to that described in the "Deciding to Make the Change" section of Step One (Chapter 13).

It could be difficult for you to decide to stop purging. You may have been under the impression that purging is a quick fix, a harmless way to control your body weight and shape and/or manage your mood. However, it is important you know that self-induced vomiting is not an effective means of controlling weight, as you only sick up part of what you ate. Laxatives and diuretics do not eliminate calories at all—only water. If you are low weight, it is vital that you decide to stop purging when you decide to tackle weight restoration.

Think about the importance of stopping these behaviours. Consider whether self-induced vomiting and/or the misuse of laxatives and diuretics gives you something positive you are afraid of losing. But reflect too on the short- and long-term effects of these behaviours on your physical health, psychological functioning, interpersonal relationships and school/work performance. Wouldn't it be nice to free yourself and recover from your eating disorder? At the end of this process, you should reach a conclusion about whether or not you want to tackle your purging behaviour(s). Write it under your pros and cons table.

Strategies and procedures for tackling purging

The best strategy for stopping laxative misuse will depend on how you use them. If you take them every now and then, it is best to go "cold turkey." If, on the other hand, you take them all the time, you should wean yourself off them gradually. Your therapist will help you draw up a schedule—say halving the dose each week—and manage any issues that come up. When you stop taking laxatives or while they are being phased out, rebound fluid retention may cause you to experience a week or so of weight gain. Be aware of this possibility, and don't panic if it happens. Your therapist will help you to cope with any temporary swelling and any weight gain due to water retention.

The main procedures adopted by CBT-E to address purging for weight control are the following:

- *Self-monitoring purging in real time.* Notice the events, thoughts, and emotions that you experience before you purge and write them down in real time in the "Context and Comments" column of your monitoring record. If you do this before you start purging, it will make you more aware of what you are doing, thinking and feeling at the precise time that the urge to purge strikes. This information should help you identify triggers and make it easier for you to resist doing it.
- *Tackling the urge to purge.* As with tackling the urge to binge, the procedure "thing to say and things to do" (see Step One) may help you ride out the urge to purge (urge surfing). The trick is to do something that makes purging less likely.

If you use purging for other reasons, you can use the following specific procedures to tackle it:

- *Purging to modulate mood.* If you use vomiting to cope with strong emotions, you should use the procedures in the Events, Moods and Eating module described in Chapter 21.
- *Purging to stop feeling full.* If you vomit to avoid feeling full, you should use the procedures in the Low Weight and Undereating module discussed in Chapter 16.
- *Purging to make the stomach appear flatter.* If you take laxatives to empty out your gut so that your stomach looks flat when lying down, it is important to know that laxative misuse has little or no effect on the number of calories you absorb. Temporary gut emptying has no permanent effect on body shape.

Annie's story

I stopped eating so much when I was 14 and some mean girls at school laughed at me for being "dumpy." My mom and pop told me to ignore them, that they were just jealous of my curves, but I couldn't. I started hiding my food in my lap at mealtimes instead of eating it and my weight got really low. My parents found me out and watched me while I ate, and my weight went up, so I started throwing up after every meal I could. My parents found out about that too, so they sent me to CBT-E. The therapist was nice, and asked me what I was worried about, and I told her I was worried about getting fat because I didn't want to be teased. She asked me about my eating habits, and I told her about the hiding food and vomiting, and that I would only eat diet food that I made myself. I didn't want to eat anything my mom made because it might be fattening. She asked me if I counted calories and I said yes, and I sometimes just smell food or chew it and spit it out. I told her that I tried to lose weight by exercising, too, as well as being sick after meals. I got that this was not a great idea, but I thought it was the best way to lower my weight.

It wasn't too difficult for me to stick to regular eating, but I still threw up at least once or twice a day. My therapist drew a picture on a piece of paper to show me that this was making my eating disorder worse, and told me about all the harm that this could do. She explained that being sick after eating does not get rid of all the calories, and that there are better ways to keep my weight under control. She told me that if I felt the urge to be sick after meals, I should do something else to take my mind off it for a while. She said that urges are like waves, they get bigger and smaller, and I should try to surf them until they pass. I love getting my nails painted and making necklaces, so I got my mom to help me do these after meals. This really helped and it was nice that my parents stopped being so suspicious of me all the time.

In summary

If you use vomiting and/or misuse laxatives as a routine form of weight control, you will be encouraged to do the Purging module.

Purging needs to be addressed for the following reasons:

- It is harmful to your health.
- It requires secrecy and deception and produces feelings of guilt.
- It is only partially effective (vomiting) or ineffective (laxatives and diuretics) at eliminating the calories you take in.
- It makes binge-eating more likely because it gives you a false sense of security. You relax control of your diet, thinking incorrectly that you can "cancel out" any food you eat by making yourself sick or taking laxatives.

You must decide to stop purging after weighing up the pros and cons of doing so with your therapist. Then, to help you, you can use the following CBT-E procedures:

- Real-time self-monitoring of purging
- Tackling the urge to purge with "things to say and do"

• Take-home message

Purging is harmful and does not help you control your weight. It makes sense to stop now.

19

Body Image module

The Body Image module is designed to help you tackle your overvaluation of shape, weight and their control. It will help you learn to judge your self-worth on things other than your shape, weight and ability to control them. As we talked about in Chapter 3, the overvaluation of shape, weight and their control is the central, or "core," psychological problem in most eating disorders. It is directly or indirectly responsible for most of the other expressions of your eating disorder. You restrict your diet because you overvalue your shape and weight, you exercise excessively because you overvalue your shape and weight, you are preoccupied with food because you overvalue your shape and weight and so on. This is why your overvaluation occupies a central place in your formulation and why it is one of the most important targets of treatment. Indeed, unless you successfully overcome it, you are at considerable risk of relapse.

Addressing your overvaluation of shape and weight will take time. Changing the way you think is a gradual process. Therefore, if you are not low weight, starting this work early in Step Two is best. However, if you have a low weight, the Body Image module is usually implemented when you regain a certain amount of weight, or at the start of Step Two if you have shape and weight concerns that are making it difficult to regain weight.

The CBT-E strategies that you will use for addressing your concerns about body image are as follows:

- Drawing a pie chart of your self-evaluation system
- Creating an extended personal formulation of your eating disorder
- Enhancing the importance of other self-evaluation domains
- Tackling shape checking and shape avoidance
- Tackling feeling fat

Remember that the overvaluation of shape and weight is not the same as body dissatisfaction. Overvaluation is more closely linked to self-esteem than body dissatisfaction. People without an eating disorder may be dissatisfied with their bodies, but it doesn't take over their lives.

DOI: 10.4324/9781003342489-21

Drawing your self-evaluation system pie chart

As we have seen, most people judge themselves based on their success in several areas of life that they consider important. In young people, common self-evaluation domains are relationships with family members and friends, school or work achievements, sports and other activities. They may be given different levels of importance, but they all factor into how you see yourself. There may also be domains that are generally thought to be important—your grades, for example—but do not, in fact, influence how you feel about your self-worth. The easy way to tell how important a life domain is to you is to imagine how you would feel if you failed in that department. If you didn't pass an exam, would it crush you, or would you just shrug it off? If someone feels very bad for a long time when an aspect of their life is not working, this is likely to be an important area of their self-evaluation. Here are two examples to explain this concept:

- If a boy judges himself based on his academic success, when he gets a low grade, he tends to overreact—he gets very upset and remains in a low mood for weeks. Contrast this with a more usual reaction to a bad grade: "Oh dear! I should have studied harder. I'll have to do better next time."
- If a girl places great importance on her relationships with others, she feels good when she is appreciated, sought out and involved in activities by her peers, but very sad or frustrated when she receives criticism or perceives disinterest from others. She gets disproportionately upset when a friend can't come out, thinking "She must hate me," rather than the more balanced and more likely to be true, "She must be busy."

In the same way, if you overvalue shape or weight, if you think you look fat or weigh too much, you feel worthless. It conditions the way you see yourself because it is the most important thing in your life.

After checking that you understand this, your therapist will encourage you to come up with a written list of the things that could affect you in this way. What things in your life would make you feel terrible if they weren't going well for you? These are your major self-evaluation domains. By the way, if you haven't added shape, weight and their control to your list, add it now.

The next thing to do is to assess how important each of these domains is to your self-evaluation system. Would falling out with a friend upset you more than getting a bad grade or less? Rank the items on your list, starting with number 1 for the most important to you, and then number 2 for the next most important and so on, until you have ranked them all.

Once you have ranked the items, you can draw a pie chart to illustrate your self-evaluation scheme. Your therapist will help you to do this, but there's no harm in practising. As we discussed in Chapter 3, the larger each slice in your

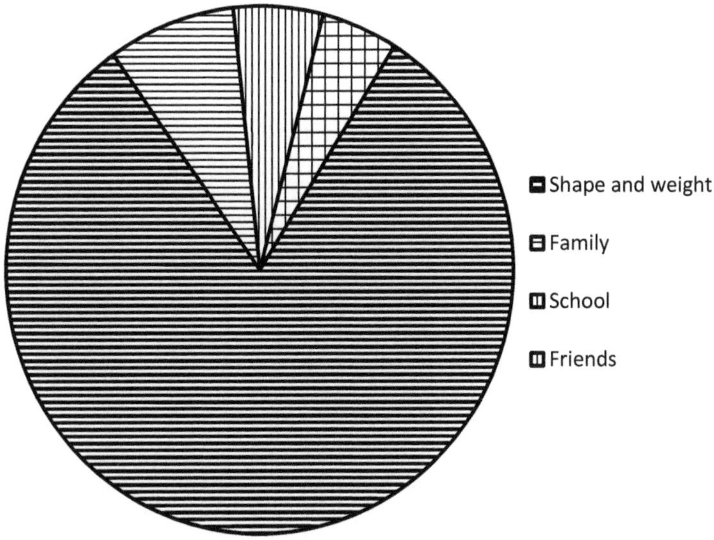

Figure 19.1 An example of a pie chart drawn up by Silvia, showing just how important her shape and weight have become to her

pie chart, the more important you think that domain is. Generally, people with eating disorders have a pie chart with a few small slices (two or three minor self-evaluation domains) and a massive slice (that of shape and weight), as shown in the example drawn up by Silvia (Figure 19.1).

The pie chart you draw is provisional, and during Step Two, you should see how your self-evaluation is progressing by redrawing your pie chart on the back of your monitoring record once a week. The goal of this module is for you to develop a more balanced self-evaluation scheme and therefore a pie chart with more similar-sized slices. No life domain should have the power to run your life—it is your job to share it out equally.

What's wrong with my uneven pie chart?

Don't get me wrong: a pie chart with a few small slices and one enormous one can seem a good idea in the short term. It is easier to for you judge yourself in one domain and it gives you a feeling of being in control. Especially at the beginning, when you first start to diet, you may have some success, which will make you feel good about yourself. Lots of smaller slices representing academic achievements, relationships, interests, sports performance, personal qualities and others can seem more difficult to manage. However, there are several unwanted effects of judging yourself mainly or only on one domain, for instance:

- *Having a pie chart with a dominant slice is risky*. A self-evaluation system of this type works well if things are going well. However, when something goes wrong in the control of shape and weight, as this is the main domain, this will inevitably lead to the whole self-evaluation system collapsing. Remember the stool with one big leg and a few little stubby legs—how long will it be able to stay upright? When you inevitably fail to meet your expectations, you will judge yourself negatively overall, as the other domains will be too small to make up for perceived failure in this one. In other words, it's like putting all your eggs in one basket.
- *Judging yourself based on your appearance and weight, and your ability to control them is doomed to failure*. The problem is not only one of having most of your eggs in one basket, because the basket you have placed your eggs in has a giant hole in the bottom. Sooner rather than later, all your eggs are going to fall out. Judging your self-worth on your ability to control your shape and weight is problematic for several reasons. The first is that your shape and weight are not under your control in the first place. What is mainly determined by your genes cannot be changed through will power. Furthermore, there are always going to be people who seem more attractive. This is partly because people with eating disorders tend to consider themselves less attractive than others, and partly because they have a skewed way of comparing themselves to others. Last but not least, judging yourself on shape and weight causes you to do things that can hurt you, and these maintain the eating disorder.
- *Focusing on one dominant slice makes it difficult to have a well-rounded, happy life*. Being concerned almost exclusively with your shape, weight and their control pushes out or marginalises other areas of life. This reduces your interests to your body alone. Because you are only interested in your shape and weight, you will neglect other interests you could have or used to have. Your relationships will crumble, your grades will fall, and, worst of all, you will have no avenues of escape. If you don't make time for other important life domains, like relationships and hobbies, you will be creating yourself a prison, where you will remain trapped with your sense of failure. To develop a functional, stable and well-rounded self-evaluation system, you need to extend your areas of interest.

Creating your extended personal formulation

Once you have drawn up your pie chart, the next step is to create your *extended personal formulation*. This is a personal formulation that illustrates the *consequences* of your overvaluation of shape, weight and their control. With the help of your therapist, you will analyse what you do or experience as a result of the importance you place on your shape, weight and their control. In general, the most common consequences are the following:

- Marginalisation of other areas of life
- Body checking
- Body avoidance
- Feeling fat

For practice, think about whether you have experienced any of these consequences of the overvaluation of shape and weight in the last four weeks. Write those that do apply to you in the boxes in Figure 19.2. All you need to do is go over the light grey writing with a darker pen. Below the "Strict dieting" box, you should include the behaviours you identified in your provisional personal formulation during Step One (see Figure 8.2 in Chapter 8) if they still apply.

Then you can draw your extended personal formulation in pencil on a blank sheet of paper. You should put this in the ring binder that you use to store your monitoring records. Look at the extended personal formulation in Figure 19.3. This was drawn up by William and shows the eating-disorder features he identified at the beginning and how they interact with each other.

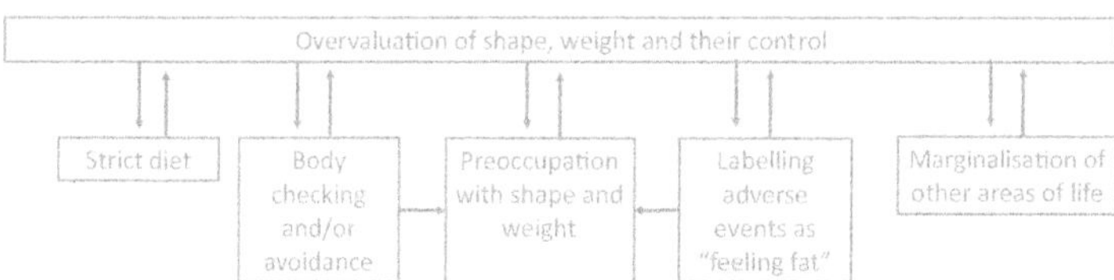

Figure 19.2 Diagram with empty boxes you can use to build your own extended personal formulation – go over the boxes and arrows that apply to you

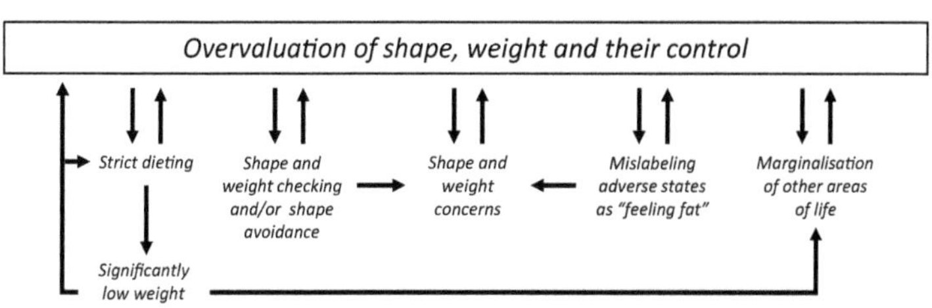

Figure 19.3 An example of an extended personal formulation drawn up by William; his shape checking and avoidance fuel his overvaluation, and he tends to equate feeling fat with being fat, which intensifies his shape and weight concerns

Two-prong strategy for tackling overvaluation

To develop a more functional self-evaluation scheme, you need to attack it from both sides. We suggest that you apply two complementary strategies:

1. *Enhancing the importance of other life domains*. This will involve doing new things to increase the number and size of other slices in your pie chart.
2. *Reducing the importance of shape, weight and their control*. You can reduce the size of your "shape and weight" slice by directly tackling the things your overvaluation of shape and weight makes you do, like shape checking, shape avoidance and/or feeling fat.

Enhancing the importance of other life domains

The goal is to begin focusing more on other aspects of life so that these things become more important slices in your self-evaluation pie chart. You should make a conscious effort to engage more in your other life domains, such as school activities, work, your social life and hobbies, to give these a chance to grow. You should also try out new things to see if they could become new slices. Look on this as a wonderful opportunity to experiment. It should also help you deal with things that you have shelved because of your eating disorder, to become more independent and to complete your psychological and social development.

There are three steps to enhancing the importance of other life domains. Your therapist will discuss them with you and help you put them into practice:

1. *Identify new activities that you might be interested in doing*. Think about your interests and activities before the onset of the eating disorder and/or new things you might like to try. Sometimes good ideas can come from considering what your friends do outside school.
2. *Decide on one or two activities that you will try out*. It may be helpful you involve your friends or siblings in this process, as you will be more likely to stick with an activity if you are doing with someone. Make a date to go to a tango lesson or to get your nails done. Not only should this be fun, it will also give you a chance to work on your interpersonal skills.
3. *Review your progress week by week*. You should use the proactive problem-solving procedure described in Chapter 22 to overcome any difficulties you might experience as you are trying to expand your sphere of interests. Note that there is no point in flogging a dead horse. If you try an activity and don't like it, do something else! As a rule of thumb, if you don't click with something after three tries, forget about it and pick a new activity. Towards the end of treatment, you should redraw your pie chart. This will give you an opportunity to review your progress. The slice representing your shape and weight should have shrunk in size to make way for the new slices.

Tackling shape checking

It is common for teenagers to check their body to some extent, but many young people with eating disorders repeatedly do so, often in an unusual way. Because body checking tends to be particularly influential in maintaining dissatisfaction with shape and prompting dieting, as described in Chapter 3, it is best to address this aspect of body image first.

In Step One, during in-session weighing, you will have already tackled one form of body checking: weight checking. You probably find in-session weighing helpful, as it will have lessened your concerns about weight and your fixation with the number on the scales. In a similar way, tackling shape checking can reduce your concerns about shape. As with weight checking, you may experience an increase in your concerns about your shape when you start to try to get to grips with shape checking, but this will only be short-lived.

The procedure we to address shape checking has five main steps:

1. *Identifying the various forms of your shape checking.* Shape checking can become a habit, and you may not be fully aware that you are doing it. You may automatically compare yourself with others you see while walking down the street without even realising. This is why you should record your shape checking in real time in detail for two 24-hour periods. You can use an adaptation of the usual monitoring record for this purpose. The adapted monitoring record should include the columns "Check" for you to write when and how long you checked your shape and "Place" for you to note where you did it. One of these monitoring days should be a school or work day, and the other a day off school or work.

There is a blank monitoring record for shape checking (Table 28.2) in the CBT-E TOOLS at the back of this book. Your therapist will provide you with one of your own, but if you want to practice you can photocopy the one in this book or download it using the QR code:

These are common forms of shape checking. If you answer yes to any of these questions, you should write them down on your monitoring record:

- Do you spend ages looking at certain parts of your body in the mirror with an overcritical attitude?
- Do you flex your muscles to see how big they are several times a day?

- Is it impossible for you to pass a reflective surface without checking out your belly, thighs, abs or butt?
- Do you check the size and shape of your stomach or thighs when sitting down?
- Do you check if there is a space between the tops of your thighs when you press them together?
- Do you measure your waist, hips, thighs, wrists or other body parts using a tape measure?
- Do you place a ruler on your hip bones to see if it there is a space underneath, where your belly is?
- Do you pinch or touch parts of your body to see how big or small they are?
- Do you prod yourself to see if you can feel your bones or muscles?
- Do you wear tight clothes to see how they feel?
- Do you compare yourself with people who are thinner or have features you admire (like a flat belly, big muscles or long, slim legs)?
- Do you follow models or actors of the same sex in the media and on social media because you would like to look like them?
- Do you ask other people or wonder about their weight or body measurements?
- Do you fish for compliments about your body shape?

The real-time monitoring of shape checking is intended to help you become aware of all your checking behaviours, and how these affect your concerns about body shape.

2. *Weighing up your reasons for and the consequences of body checking*. The next step will be to discuss with your therapist why you check your shape so often, and what effects this has. As part of this discussion, you should respond to the following questions:

   - "What are you trying to find out when you check your body? Do you really think you can find it out this way?" If you are trying to find out what your shape is like, you are going about it the wrong way. Constantly looking at yourself or pinching, prodding or measuring yourself tends to magnify your "imperfections" and make you think that some aspects of body shape that are normal, like having rounded stomach, are not. If, on the other hand, you are trying to reassure yourself that your shape is changing and you are not getting fat, you should reflect on the fact that checking body shape does not provide reliable information, only inaccurate impressions, because you likely do not have a photographic memory. For example, when you look in the mirror, you might think you see differences between how you look in the morning and how you look in the afternoon. This is not possible and therefore cannot be accurate.
   - "Why are you checking yourself so frequently? Do you think you might be checking yourself too often?" If you are checking that your shape hasn't

changed, think about whether your shape can change so quickly. It can't, so why are you expecting it to do so? The body's shape cannot change within a few hours without significant changes in water weight. If a change in the shape of the belly is your concern, you should always bear in mind that your stomach may look rounder after eating, but this is normal, and only temporary. The same goes for muscles: they might look pumped up after a workout, but this is because they are full of blood. Do you think that having food in your belly is the same thing as putting on weight?

- "Do you ever focus on the parts of your body you like?" If not, you should ask yourself why not. Wouldn't it be a good idea to admire your hair or your hands sometimes to improve your acceptance of your own body?
- "Do you feel better after checking your body?" We can almost guarantee that the answer to this one is no. When you first began to lose weight and you checked your body only infrequently, you probably felt proud of the results you had achieved. However, by now you are probably checking yourself several times a day and expecting to see results that cannot possibly be there. Reflect on why shape checking fails to make you feel better, and probably makes you feel worse. Can you see how this behaviour maintains and intensifies your concerns about body shape? If your body checking still reassures you because it reminds you that you are thin, remember that the result of this is to fuel your eating disorder by continuing your preoccupation with your body shape.
- "Do you think your body checking has any adverse effects?" If you are not aware that shape checking has numerous negative consequences, you should know that shape checking is unhelpful for the following reasons:

    - It maintains concern about the body shape because you only, and constantly, study the parts of your body that you don't like.
    - It makes even the most attractive people find "flaws" in their body, as what we see in the mirror depends mainly on how we see ourselves.
    - It makes apparent defects look worse, because we tend to focus on what we don't like rather than looking at the bigger picture. Consequently, we have no reference points for size or scale.

3. *Categorising the various forms of shape checking*. With your therapist, you should put the forms of checking you have identified in one of two categories:

    a. *Those best stopped altogether*. These will include:

        - *Abnormal forms of behaviour*. Anything that people don't normally do, like pinching parts of your body to assess "fatness," repeatedly touching your stomach, thighs or arms, feeling your bones, checking the tightness of rings and watchstraps, looking down when sitting to see how much your belly bulges out over your waistband or how far your thighs spread.

- *Anything secretive, which would be embarrassing if someone else found out.* Whether you use a tape measure to check your thigh circumference, whether you check the gap between your thighs or place a ruler across your hip bones to check that your abdomen doesn't touch it, it doesn't matter. If you would be mortified if someone walked in on you doing it, it needs to go.

b. *Those best modified.* These are things that people normally do, but that you do to excess, like looking in a mirror, or checking out how other people look. It would in any case be impossible to stop doing these things, but you do need to work to bring them down to normal levels.

4. *Stopping abnormal forms of shape checking.* In order for you to stop shape checking, you need to become aware that you are doing it in real time. It shouldn't be too difficult for you to stop abnormal forms of shape checking, so our suggestion is that it is best to go "cold turkey" rather than trying to phase these behaviours out. Shape checking tends to undermine self-respect and, after a few weeks, you should find stopping it a relief. Just like reducing the frequency of weight checking in Step One, modifying habitual shape checking behaviour usually results in a short-lived increase in your preoccupation. However, this will soon be followed by a dramatic reduction in these thoughts and concerns. In the meantime, if you are finding it difficult to stop yourself doing certain forms of shape checking (like pinching parts of the body to assess "fatness"), you may need to do something else with your hands for a while, like playing with a fidget spinner or squeezing a ball.
5. *Modifying normal forms of shape checking.* You need to become aware of the behaviour in real time, and then learn to think first before checking. Ask yourself the same questions that the therapist asks you when reviewing your shape checking monitoring records. Remind yourself that your shape could not possibly have changed since you last checked, and all that you are doing is fuelling your eating disorder. Practising this strategy will make you better at interpreting what you experience and help you gain control over your behaviour.

Cutting down on mirror use

What you see in the mirror depends on what you look at and how. Are you looking at your whole body, or just certain parts of it? Are you just giving yourself a brief glance or really examining yourself? The way you look at yourself will influence what you see and how you feel about it. Your mood will also have an impact on your self-image: when we are sad or in a bad mood, we generally feel we look worse than when we are cheerful or in a good mood. All you are doing by continually looking in the mirror is giving yourself bad data about the way you look, and at the same time increasing your preoccupation with your body shape. That is why it is important for you to cut back on your mirror use. This can be done by working through the three steps outlined next with your therapist.

1. *Assessing how you use mirrors*. Think about:
   - *How often you look in the mirror*. Look at your body checking monitoring records and consider your mirror use at home and school or work. You should monitor your mirror use from now on.
   - *How you look in the mirror*. This can be assessed by answering the following questions:
     - How long do you spend looking in the mirror each time?
     - What exactly are you checking? Which parts are you looking at and which are you ignoring or avoiding?
     - What exactly are you trying to find out?
2. *Learning about mirrors and how our way of looking in them can influence our self-image*. The image you see in the mirror does not reflect the real size of your body. If you have any doubts on this score, ask a friend to mark the top and bottom of your reflection on a full-length mirror when your whole body is reflected. How far back do you have to stand to see yourself entirely? Although you had not probably realised this, you will now see that your mirror image is 50% of the actual size. Therefore, you must be careful about how you interpret what you see when you look in a mirror.
   What you see is also influenced by *how* you look in the mirror. For example, **scrutiny** magnifies perceived defects—if you look for bulges, you will find them. Moreover, scrutinising your body for a long time without taking in reference points for scale makes you think you look bigger than you actually are. The opposite happens with fleeting reflection. For example, one of our young patients told us she accidentally caught sight of herself in a shop window and did not immediately recognise herself. Her first glance showed her as she truly is, and her negative opinion only kicked in when she realised it was *her* reflection that she was looking at.

> JARGON BUSTER
>
> **scrutiny** (noun): careful examination of something in order to get information about it—examining with an agenda

3. *Modifying your mirror use.* Here are three general questions and suggestions for correctly using the mirror:

   - *When is it appropriate to use the mirror?* Appropriate use may include checking your hair and clothing, applying or removing make-up and/or shaving.
   - *What forms of mirror use are inappropriate or unhelpful?* Examples of inappropriate mirror use include focusing on body parts you aren't happy with and scrutinising them for abnormally long periods of time.
   - *How can you avoid magnifying your apparent defects?* To avoid this effect, you should not focus on body parts that you dislike and instead look at the whole body, including more neutral areas (e.g., hands, feet, knees, hair). In addition, you should take in the background environment, as this will help give you a sense of scale.

In other words, you should modify your mirror use using two main strategies:

1. Questioning yourself before looking in the mirror and doing real-time self-monitoring
2. Changing the way you look at yourself in the mirror

The goal is to adjust your behaviour and become more skilled in interpreting what you see. It is not necessary to avoid mirrors entirely, but you should only look in the mirror for the purposes listed earlier, at least for the meantime.

You should also assess how much time you spend choosing what to wear before going out, and if you have difficulty deciding on an outfit. Suppose you spend a long time in front of a mirror, unable to choose between several outfits. This will probably make you feel gradually sadder and more dissatisfied with your shape. You may even give up on the idea of going out altogether because you don't think you look good in anything. If you find yourself in this situation, next time commit to an outfit before you put it on. Do not get dressed in front of a mirror.

Addressing comparison making

Repeated *comparison making* is a particular form of body checking that actively maintains concerns about shape. Usually, there are two forms of comparison making: (1) comparing yourself with other people and (2) comparing yourself with images in the media.

The result of comparison making is generally for you to conclude that your own body is less attractive than those you have chosen to compare it with. This is because your view is biased in one, or both, of two ways:

1. You chose thin and attractive people, not others who are less slim and worse-looking than you, to compare yourself with. This is an example of

subject bias—what you are comparing yourself with is unfair. Think about a local team trying to take on a national team—they may be top of their own league, but they are highly unlikely to win against the big stars. It would not be a fair match.

2. You look at their bodies quickly and uncritically. This is very different to the way you look at yourself: for long periods of time and focusing on the bits you don't like. This is an example of *assessment bias*—how you are comparing yourself is unfair. Think about judging a gymnastics performance. If you judged one gymnast on what you saw in the moment and another using a video replayed over and over, looking for the flaws, that would hardly be fair, would it?

In order to stop these unhelpful forms of comparison, your therapist will help you attack them from both sides, by:

1. *Addressing subject bias*. You need to start noticing that you only compare yourself with extremely attractive people, and draw the logical conclusions from this awareness. To this end, your therapist will encourage you to conduct the following experiment:

   a. Walk along a street, compare yourself with every third person of your age and gender, and then reflect on what you discover. You will almost certainly notice that people are far more varied in appearance than you had previously noticed, and some people with body shapes that you consider "unattractive" actually look pretty good. Reflect also on the notion of "attractiveness," which is not only related to thinness. Broaden your comparison making to include aspects of people other than their shape. Take into account their hair, shoes, sense of humour and so on.

2. *Addressing assessment bias*. To get a handle on the assessment bias underlying your comparison making, your therapist will encourage you to conduct another experiment:

   a. Go into a shared changing room, for example at a swimming pool, have a quick look round and find someone you think looks good. Without them noticing, furtively scrutinise that person's body, focusing on the parts you dislike about your own body, and then reflect on what you find. Bodies that appear attractive at first glance likely have flaws and imperfections if you examine them more carefully.

In recent years, comparing ourselves with people portrayed in the media has become common. If you do this sort of thing, you should monitor this form of comparison making, which might include images from social media, the internet and/or magazines. Try not to uncritically accept what you see in the media, and research body image manipulation (airbrushing and similar). You may also find these two videos helpful:

1. Evolution—www.youtube.com/watch?v=iYhCn0jf46U
2. Real beauty sketches—www.youtube.com/watch?v=litXW91UauE

Try to cut back on looking at fashion magazines or watching TV programmes featuring images of slim women (fashion, beauty contests, etc.). Remember that the beauties they star are the equivalent of world-class athletes—if they were boxers, there is no way you would step in the ring with them, and you wouldn't feel bad about yourself for refusing to fight. These people are likely in the media precisely because they are so attractive. Comparing yourself with them would not be a fair fight. Take it to heart too that pro-ana sites are not your friends—they only encourage preoccupation with shape and weight, and fan the flames of your eating disorder. If your friends made you feel as bad as these things make you feel, would you get rid of them or let them stick around?

Tackling body avoidance

Some people with eating disorders avoid looking at their bodies and dislike other people looking at them. Often these people have engaged in repeated body checking in the past but have switched over to body avoidance because body checking became too distressing.

Shape avoidance may take the form of avoiding looking in the mirror, not wearing tight clothes, covering the stomach (with loose clothing or a cushion when seated) and not looking at photographs of yourself.

Why is shape avoidance bad?

Shape avoidance needs to be addressed directly because it is a major spoke in the wheel of your recovery. As described in Chapter 3, it maintains your concerns about your body shape because without objective data, your fears will dictate how you feel. You will think that you look worse than you do and will be prompted to use dietary restraint and other extreme weight-control behaviours. Moreover, it will prevent you from socialising, being physically intimate with your partner, swimming, using public changing rooms or buying new clothes. Therefore, if you practice shape avoidance you need to take back control.

You have already addressed one form of body avoidance, namely weight avoidance, in Step One during in-session weighing. Just as knowing what you actually weigh made you less concerned about what you might weigh, knowing what you actually look like will dispel your fears about what you think you look like. Remember that focusing on shape avoidance might increase your shape concerns for a while, but this will only be a temporary state of affairs—a hump you need to get over in order to feel better about yourself.

How will CBT-E help me tackle shape avoidance?

The first thing to do is to confirm that you do it. This is generally relatively simple, as you are probably already aware of doing it. You know that you don't like to look at yourself or have others look at you. Usually, it exists on a spectrum, ranging from minor sensitivity to seeing your body or others seeing it to total shape avoidance. You should think about why you wear baggy clothes. Is it just your style, or is related to your shape concerns? If you are having trouble working this out, ask yourself questions like these:

- What kind of clothes do your friends wear?
- Is baggy the "in" thing?
- Did you also avoid wearing better-fitting clothes before the onset of your eating disorder?
- If not, why did you change your style?
- Would you be able to wear tighter clothes than usual to go to a party?

Getting over your shape avoidance will involve gradual exposure therapy. Just as if you were scared of snakes or dogs, you would be gradually exposed to them in a safe place, from just being in the same room with them to touching or stroking them, until you have conquered your fear. Your therapist will help you first to recognise your shape avoidance, and then to plan specific body exposure "experiments," beginning with situations that will create the smallest discomfort.

The goal is for you to understand that wearing loose clothing, as well as other forms of body avoidance, is not a free choice but is dictated by your eating disorder mindset. You need to gradually get used to the sight and feel of your body. You need to get used to others seeing your body, too. You must stop dressing and undressing in the dark and wearing shapeless, baggy clothes. You also need to get accustomed to using mirrors (bearing in mind the information in the section on mirror use earlier) and participating in normal activities that involve body exposure, such as swimming or going to the beach.

Some examples of shape avoidance and how to gradually address them are as follows:

- *Avoiding others seeing your body*. If you avoid wearing tight or revealing clothes:
    - o Start by wearing less baggy, shapeless clothes.
    - o Work towards being able to wear more form-fitting clothes, including swimming costumes.

- *Avoiding being touched.* If you flinch when someone comes close:
    - o Start by asking a trusted friend or parent to pat or hug you—whomever or whatever you feel safest with.
    - o Work towards being able to be touched by other friends and romantic partners.

And in extreme situations:

- *Avoiding the sight of your body.* If you only get dressed and undressed in the dark:
    - o Start by getting dressed and undressed by candlelight.
    - o Work towards getting dressed and undressed with the light on and the curtains open.
- *Avoiding touching your body.* If you try to wash yourself without touching yourself:
    - o Wash in a self-aware way, using your bare hands and starting with body parts that don't offend you (perhaps your feet, forearms or hands). Apply body lotion to the same areas.
    - o Work towards being able to wash your whole body with your hands and apply body lotion all over.

Make sure that you don't go overboard and swap body avoidance for repeated body checking, which is always a risk. That would be like jumping out of the frying pan and into the fire. What you are aiming for is a happy medium. It is normal to check your shape when you try on a new outfit or get dressed in the morning, and that's where you want to be.

Tackling feeling fat

Feeling fat is an experience that many people have, but the intensity and frequency of this feeling appear to be far greater if you have an eating disorder. This is a problem because you likely equate feeling fat with being fat. This is true of both underweight and not underweight people. It is an expression of excessive concern about shape and weight, but it also maintains it, reinforcing shape dissatisfaction and prompting dieting, so it needs to be addressed.

Feeling fat fluctuates daily and throughout the day, while body shape barely changes within such a short timeframe. Therefore, something else is likely responsible for these fluctuations in feelings of fatness. As described in Chapter 3, feeling fat appears to result from you mislabelling other experiences, for example:

- *Body awareness.* Comments on your appearance, body checking, physical contact, being sweaty, your bits wobbling and tight clothing may all make you feel fat, but that doesn't mean that you are. That would be like saying "I am, therefore I'm fat."

- *Adverse physical states*. Feeling bloated, premenstrual, full, hungover or sleepy may also make you feel fat, but they are not the same thing at all.
- *Adverse emotional states*. Likewise for feeling depressed, lonely, bored or unloved.

To help you get over these feelings it is clear that something needs to be done. You cannot go through life feeling fat every time something unpleasant happens, so you need to find better ways of dealing with these sensations.

How will CBT-E help me get over feeling fat?

In general, working on feeling fat is best left until you have reduced your body checking and/or body avoidance because these behaviours may be triggers for feeling fat. However, this is not always the right approach. If feeling fat is particularly prominent or distressing for you, your therapist may reverse the order and ask you to address it first.

The strategy is for you to identify the experiences that trigger feeling fat and tackle them directly. If you apply this strategy over time, you will no longer equate feeling fat with being fat, and it will cease to maintain your eating disorder. The strategy includes three steps:

1. *Noticing the feeling*. As soon as you feel fat, write it in the Comments column of your monitoring record.
2. *Identifying their triggers*. Immediately after each peak, ask yourself the following two questions:
   - Has anything happened in the last hour that might have triggered my feeling fat?
   - What else am I feeling just now (besides fat)?
3. *Addressing the triggers directly*. Here are some examples of triggers you may have identified and how best to cope with them:
   - *You feel fat because you checked your body in the mirror*. Tell yourself you will only look in the mirror in the morning before going outside, not to scrutinise the body parts that you don't like.
   - *You feel fat because you're wearing tight clothes*. Decide to wear more comfortable clothes.
   - *You feel fat because you're tired*. Take a nap.
   - *You feel fat because you feel lonely*. Call a friend and invite them out for a walk.

Over time, the frequency and intensity of feeling fat generally gradually wanes, and you become able to stop equating it with being fat. Once this happens, feeling fat loses its power to maintain your shape concerns.

Margaret's story

I've never been very self-confident, and I worried about my weight a lot. I do rhythmic gymnastics and I wanted to be in the best possible shape, so I started cutting calories. I thought I'd get better at my sport and like myself more. However, the more weight I lost, the more worried I got about my body shape. By the time I got help I was weighing myself several times a day and I'd spend hours in front of a mirror, pinching my fat bits and feeling bad about myself. I agreed to see a therapist because I had zero energy. I wasn't worried about the weight I'd lost, but my periods had stopped, and I had gotten really weak, meaning I had difficulty keeping up with training.

The treatment they got me was CBT-E, which went fine until we got to the part when I had to try to put on weight. This made me even more worried about getting fat and what I looked like, so I basically failed at that. My therapist asked me if I thought looking in the mirror and weighing myself all the time reassured me or made me more worried, and after thinking about it for a while I said it made me more worried. She said that this was normal, and showed me the ways that constant "body checking," as she called it, makes the eating disorder worse, because it doesn't give you chance to think about anything positive. You are always just standing there, hating yourself. She said that my body image seemed to be a problem for me, and because it was making it difficult for me to eat properly, we should do something about it straight away. That's when we started the Body Image module, which wasn't easy, but helped me stop poking and prodding at myself all the time and get over my obsession with how I looked.

I didn't have to change my behaviour straight away—the first week I spent two days monitoring my body checking. This made me realise just how much I was doing it—I was spending more time doing that than I was doing anything else! My therapist seemed quite pleased with how well I had completed this task, and we talked for a while about how body checking was affecting my life and my moods, and that I wasn't being fair to myself. She got me to agree to reduce each of my checking behaviours, one at a time, and to see what effect this would have. The next week I made a real effort to stop touching my hip bones and fat bits. To be honest, after a few days it wasn't so hard to do. This gave me the confidence to try to cut down on mirror use in the next week and so on. No longer spending so much time checking my body made me worry less about it and gave me more time to do other things that made me feel better about myself—or at least not worse! I don't exactly love my body now, but I accept that it is the one nature gave me so it will do.

In summary

The Body Image module is applied if you experience overvaluation of shape, weight and their control—if you judge your self-worth mainly or only on these things.

The strategies that CBT-E uses for addressing concerns about body image are as follows:

- Drawing a pie chart of your self-evaluation system
- Creating an extended personal formulation
- Adopting two complementary strategies to address the overvaluation of shape and weight and their control:

1. Increasing the importance of other life domains (by increasing the size and number of slices in your self-evaluation pie chart).
2. Reducing the importance of shape, weight and their control (by decreasing the size of the "shape and weight" slice of your self-evaluation pie chart). To do this you may need to tackle the main expressions of your overvaluation—shape checking, shape avoidance and/or feeling fat, directly.

• Take-home message

Transforming your body image will take time. Changing the way you think about yourself is a gradual process, but with practice you should be able to shake off the shackles of your overvaluation and develop a healthier, more functional way of judging yourself.

Dietary Rules module

The Dietary Rules module is for helping you tackle your extreme and rigid dietary rules. You will start it a couple of weeks after the Body Image module (if you are not low weight) or during the process of weight regain with the Low Weight and Undereating module (if you are low weight).

As described in Chapter 3, it is essential to distinguish two aspects of strict dieting; these are:

1. *Dietary restriction*—not eating enough for your body's needs
2. *Dietary restraint*—attempting to limit what you eat

Dietary restriction is addressed using the procedures described in the Low Weight and Undereating module. In contrast, the Dietary Rules module tackles dietary restraint and dietary rules, alongside your overvaluation of control over eating. Your reasons for dieting, in particular your concerns about shape and weight, are addressed with the procedure described in the Body Image module.

Weighing up the pros and cons of relaxing dietary rules

Dietary rules need to be interrupted for two main reasons (see the section "Extreme Dieting" in Chapter 3 for more details):

1. They cause physical, psychological, and interpersonal harm.
2. They play a central role in maintaining eating disorders, as they may result in undereating and weight loss or low weight. As such, they also make binge-eating episodes more likely (see Chapter 3).

As with the other features of your eating disorder, you alone must make the decision to address dietary rules. It is a decision that cannot be made by your therapist or other people. However, we are aware that this decision is often

DOI: 10.4324/9781003342489-22

difficult, as you may consider some dietary rules a positive way of controlling your shape and weight. In addition, dieting is constantly portrayed as a good thing in the media. You may also be using your ability to stick to dietary rules as a measure of your willpower or to compensate for binge-eating episodes or manage excess body weight. All these things can make it hard for you to let go.

This is why it is important for you to discuss your reasons for and against change with your therapist. To help you make the decision to tackle your dietary rules, your therapist will help you draw up a pros-and-cons-of-change table, just like you did when deciding to address weight regain. If you are low weight, the two decisions go hand in hand—you cannot restore weight without relaxing your dietary rules.

First, start to list your cons. Consider whether your dietary rules provide you with benefits that you would be afraid to lose and what they might be. Then, think carefully about the advantages of changing. What are the short- and long-term effects of dietary rules on your health, psychological functioning and interpersonal relationships? The only way to free yourself from these effects and overcome your eating disorder is to change.

Don't worry about losing control over your weight if you interrupt your dietary rules. Replacing them with healthy and flexible nutritional guidelines is the best way to maintain weight control in the long term. These reflections should help you come to a conclusion. Are you going to tackle your dietary rules? If not, the programme cannot be continued.

Identifying dietary rules

In general, extreme and inflexible dietary rules concern (1) what and how much you will eat; (2) what you won't eat; and (3) what time you will/won't allow yourself to eat. You may also have other rules, such as eating a precise number of calories, not eating more than anyone else at the table or until you have earned it. Identifying your dietary rules may not be so easy, as they may have become an automatic habit. A clue to help you recognise your dietary rules are the asterisks (*) in your monitoring record. You put them there when you thought you deviated from your eating plan. What triggers your binge-eating episodes? Working this out can also be particularly revealing.

To help you become aware of your dietary rules in real time, your therapist will ask you to write them down on your monitoring record. If you are having difficulties in identifying them, think about whether you would have a problem with eating in certain situations, like at a restaurant or someone's home. Why would this be difficult for you? List the reasons.

There is also a handy questionnaire to help you identify your dietary rules. This is called the Dietary Rule Inventory (Table 28.6), and you can find it in the CBT-E TOOLS at the back of this book. If you answer any of the questions "sometimes," "often" or "always," this is probably a dietary rule that should be addressed. Your therapist will provide you with one of your own, but if you want to practice you can photocopy the one in this book or download it using the QR code:

General strategy for relaxing dietary rules

You can deal with the dietary rules you have identified with the following general strategy:

1. *Asking yourself why you have a specific dietary rule.* If you broke it, why would that worry you? Dietary rules are often motivated by the goal of losing weight or avoiding weight gain, or fear that breaking the rule would result in an episode of binge eating.
2. *Critically analysing the likely consequences of breaking the rule.* Generally speaking, breaking most dietary rules does not result in weight gain, as this depends on the amount of food you eat overall. A binge-eating episode is also unlikely to result, as this will depend on your *reaction* to breaking the rule. You feel bad because you broke the rule and you binge to make yourself feel better. If you didn't have the rule in the first place, you wouldn't be able to break it, and therefore you wouldn't feel bad. Think too about the positive consequences of adopting flexible eating guidelines instead. It would certainly make eating a lot simpler and less stressful.
3. *Breaking the rule on purpose.* Say one of your rules is not eating after 6 pm. Your therapist will ask you to decide to do so. They will help you plan what you will eat, when, where and with whom. They will also provide you with a proactive procedure for solving problems and managing the period following the rule-breaking (as described in Chapter 22).
4. *Examining the implications of breaking the rule.* Talk with your therapist about what happened and re-evaluate the concerns and beliefs you had before breaking the rule. Consider the potential advantages of adopting a more flexible approach to eating.
5. *Planning further occasions for breaking the same rule.* The therapist will continue to help you to plan these occasions as above, until breaking the rule has no particular significance for you.

If you systematically follow the strategy described, one rule at a time, your belief that sticking to strict dietary rules is necessary to prevent bingeing and putting on weight will gradually fade. By experiencing that the consequences of breaking dietary rules you feared—weight gain and binges—do not actually occur, you will gradually come to recognise that your dietary rules are a problem rather than a helpful way of controlling eating and body weight.

Tackling specific dietary rules

Rules on what to eat (aka addressing food avoidance)

The first step in tackling this rule is to always keep these three pieces of information in mind:

1. No food is inherently fattening (it depends on the quantity—a calorie is a calorie).
2. If you won't eat food whose composition you are unsure of, it is impossible to have a normal social life.
3. Knowledge of exactly what you are eating (in terms of calorie or fat content) is not necessary for successful weight control.

The second step in addressing food avoidance is taking a trip to the local supermarket or looking at an online shopping list. Come up with a list of all the foods you would be reluctant to eat. You may avoid them because you think they are fattening, or because you would be afraid of them triggering a binge-eating episode. Then, rate each avoided food from 1 to 4 based on the difficulty you would have eating them, with 1 being the least threatening and 4 the most. Make a list of all the 1s, 2s, 3s and 4s, like Jose did (see Figure 20.1).

FEAR LEVEL →

Group 1	*Group 2*	*Group 3*	*Group 4*
Corn flakes	*Grapes*	*Fried chicken*	*Cream*
Fruit ice cream	*Bananas*	*Ham*	*Cake*
Potatoes	*Avocado*	*Snacks*	*Milk chocolate*
	Sushi	*Pork*	*French fries*
	Soft cheese	*Pasta*	*Hard cheese*
		Chips	*Bacon*
		Pizza	*Oil*
		Crackers	*Sugar*
		Ice cream	*Pie*
		Hard candies	*Cookies*
		Dark chocolate	*Pastries and croissants*
		Whole Milk	*Frosting*

Figure 20.1 An example avoided food list—these are the foods that Jose has been avoiding

The next step is to gradually introduce the foods you have been avoiding into your diet. You should start with foods from the least problematic group, then gradually move up the scale. Try to introduce at least three avoided foods over the next week. Plan to eat them on the days when you feel in control. Make sure you highlight these foods on your monitoring record by writing the word "NEW" next to it. Write what happened and how it made you feel in the Comments column. Look at Jose's example in Figure 20.2.

Day Monday **Date** May 15th

Time	Foods and drink consumed	Place	*	V/L/E	Context and comments
	Today's plan				
7:00	I cup of yogurt Cereal I orange juice	Kitchen			
10:30	I apple	School bar			
13:30	Pasta with pesto Salad with oil and vinegar I slice of white bread (NEW) 2 glasses of water I orange	School canteen			
4:30	I cappuccino I croissant (NEW) I glass of water	Bar			
w7:00	I burger with white bread French fries (NEW) 2 glasses of water	Kitchen			
7:00	I cup of yogurt Cereal I orange juice	Kitchen			Usual breakfast—I feel OK
10:30	I apple	School bar			As I planned
13:30	Pasta with pesto Salad with oil and vinegar I white bread (NEW) 2 glasses of water I apple	Kitchen			This is the first time I have eaten two types of carbs together (pasta and bread). I am a little worried, but I will stick to my plan
4:30	I cappuccino I croissant (NEW) I glass of water I teaspoon of sugar (NEW)	Bar			As planned. I feel ok. I've got this! 😎
7:00	I burger French fries (NEW) 2 glasses of water	Kitchen			Well, I feel in control, but I left the burger bun. I will try to do it next time.
9:00	I cup of chamomile tea	Lounge			

Figure 20.2 An example of a monitoring record filled in by Jose, who is working on introducing avoided foods

If your list of avoided foods is very long and detailed, select one from each category as a test case, for example one type of chocolate. Success at introducing one representative food should reduce your concerns about the whole food category. If you see that one type of chocolate didn't hurt you, you will understand that the others are unlikely to also.

It is not necessary for you to eat a whole portion of the avoided food the first time you eat it. However, the ultimate goal is for you to be able to eat average amounts of these foods without difficulty, so you will need to build up as your fear diminishes. Sometimes this will take time, but the systematic introduction of avoided foods should continue until you are no longer anxious about eating them.

Rules on when to eat (or rather when not to eat)

You have already addressed these rules in Step One by introducing regular eating. Suppose you are still having difficulty regularising the frequency of your meals and snacks. In that case, bear in mind that there is no right or wrong time to eat, that there are no differences in calorie absorption if the food is eaten at different times of the day. Delaying eating only makes binge-eating episodes more likely.

Eating regularly, at maximum intervals of four hours, has many advantages:

- It provides structure to eating habits (and the day).
- It addresses one of the three forms of dieting (skipping meals—the other two are eliminating food and reducing food portions).
- It interrupts the cycle between dietary restraint and binge eating.
- It reduces the sense of early fullness that you may have if you are low weight.
- It reduces your concerns about eating.

Eating regularly only requires that you do two things:

1. Eat three meals plus two snacks a day at planned times no more than four hours apart.
2. Not eat between, using the "things to say and to do" procedure to manage any impulse to eat outside the scheduled times.

Rules on how much to eat

The "right" amount of food to eat overall is that which allows you to maintain a stable, healthy weight. This applies to daily intake, meals and portion sizes. For accepted nutritional guidelines and other helpful information, your therapist should be able to point you to a country-specific website. For example:

- Dietary Guidelines for Americans (www.health.gov)
- UK Eatwell Guide (www.nhs.uk/live-well/eat-well/food-guidelines-and-food-labels/the-eatwell-guide)

- Australian Dietary Guidelines (www.eatforhealth.gov.au/guidelines)
- Italian healthy eating guidelines (www.crea.gov.it/web/alimenti-e-nutrizione/-/linee-guida-per-una-sana-alimentazione-2018)

Rules on not eating in front of others

These rules make it impossible to function socially. They can also damage relationships. If you eat in public, you may be worrying about what others will be thinking about what or how much you are eating and judging you. Will they notice what you are eating and think you are greedy or have no control? The answer is no. The mistake you are making is assuming that everyone thinks the same way you do about eating control. In reality, other people do not pay any attention to what other people eat and, in any case, do not make these types of judgements about other people's eating habits.

Rules on not eating more than anyone else present

This dietary rule is based on the assumption that everyone should be eating the same amount at any given time. It does not take into account their age, sex, weight or metabolic rate. What have they eaten so far today? What will they eat later? You cannot know the answers to all of these questions, so you cannot be the one to judge whether they are eating the "right" amount. Eating less than an arbitrary amount is meaningless. Less than what?

Rules on not eating unless you are hungry

There is nothing special about resisting eating or eating only when you are famished. Extreme hunger is a condition that changes the way we think and act. Getting "hangry" is a thing. Delaying meals also intensifies your preoccupation with food and can lead to uncontrolled eating behaviours such as binge eating.

Rules on not eating unless you have done some exercise

The human body burns energy even when at rest. How much energy you use is depends on:

- *Your basal metabolic rate*. This is the energy used to make the vital organs of your body—your heart, lungs, nervous system, kidneys, liver, intestine, sexual organs and skin—work. About 60–75% of your the energy you expend each day (your resting energy expenditure) is used for this purpose.
- *Diet-induced thermogenesis*. When you eat, you produce heat. This takes up about 10% of your daily energy expenditure.

- *Physical exercise.* This accounts for just 15% to 30% of our energy expenditure—an amount that does not justify fasting until you have done some exercise. Putting off eating until you have exercised is also another sure-fire way to increase your preoccupation with food, and likely also your anxiety levels.

Rules on avoiding eating out

If you refuse to eat in restaurants, pizzerias and snack bars, you are not only making it impossible to have a social life, but you are also missing out on one of the great pleasures of living. Are you afraid of eating foods of unknown calorie composition, eating in front of others or both? If you avoid eating out, make a list of the social eating situations you avoid, and then start facing them step by step, beginning with those that create less anxiety, just like you did to tackle food avoidance.

Coping with dietary rule-breaking

A typical dysfunctional reaction to dietary rule-breaking is "all-or-nothing" reasoning. Here are some examples:

- You interpret breaking a dietary rule as evidence of having lost control ("I've ruined my diet") and lack of willpower ("I've failed").
- Breaking a dietary rule makes you abandon your attempts to control your eating ("I've lost control; I might as well give up").

If you tend to have reactions like these, you should start doing something about it by monitoring your all-or-nothing thinking in real time. When you catch yourself thinking like this, write it down on your monitoring record, and ask yourself what it means. This should enable you to decide what to do next. With practice, you should get better at not resorting to self-criticism and/or binge eating. Remember that control is adopting flexible dietary guidelines rather than extreme and inflexible dietary rules.

Tackling food checking

Dysfunctional checking of control over eating (aka food checking) is common in young people with eating disorders, particularly in those who are low weight. It is also frequently seen in those who tend to overvalue eating control, that is to say, they judge themselves mainly or only on their ability to control their eating. Common examples of food checking are the following:

- Counting calories repeatedly before and after eating
- Weighing food to eat repeatedly

- Checking food labels
- Making comparisons with what other people eat
- Asking others for reassurance about your diet

These behaviours must be addressed because they contribute to excessive eating concerns. What is more, they disrupt social life by making it impossible to eat outside the home. If any of these behaviours apply to you, you should address them by following the steps below:

1. *Real-time self-monitoring.* Since some of these behaviours are automatic, you may be unaware of doing them. As you did for body checking, you should monitor every episode of food checking in real time for two 24-hour periods on your monitoring record. What were you thinking when you decided to do this? How did it make you feel?
2. *Deciding which checking to stop, and which to modify.* As a general rule, you should stop doing the things that people don't normally do, and change the things that they do. Most people don't obsessively count calories, check food labels and compare what they eat with what other people eat. These are things that must go. Most people do, however, weigh food when they cook and portion their food. Think about how and why you are doing these things, and whether you could do them like everyone else does (see point 4 below).
3. *Stopping food checking.* Make an effort to become aware that you are doing food checking at the precise moment you are doing it, using real-time monitoring. Think about why you are doing it and make the decision not to, there and then. The goal is to become able to stop food checking entirely. Like tackling body checking, stopping food checking may raise your anxiety and concerns about eating temporarily, but these will gradually fade. If you are afraid to interrupt food checking due to a fear of gaining weight, know that it is unnecessary to count calories to maintain a stable weight.
4. *Modifying food checking.* Portioning food by repeatedly measuring or weighing it down to the gram intensifies your concern about minimal and insignificant variations in the quantity of food. However, it is normal to weigh ingredients when you are cooking and to serve yourself a healthy portion. You need to learn portion food by eye. Refer to the amounts usually served in restaurants, or the quantity you would serve to a friend who is not a dieter if you invited them to dinner. As a rule of thumb, the British Heart Foundation says your portion of chicken or fish should be about the same size as your hand, your portion of meat, beans, carbs and fruit the size of your palm, vegetables the size of two palms and your cheese portion the size of two fingers.

Tackling small meals and intermittent fasting

Another form of dietary restriction is only eating small meals and snacks. Intermittent fasting, when you have long gaps between meals and snacks, is a type of dietary restriction, too. In both cases, you are probably undereating, which may lead to the development of starvation symptoms due to weight loss. Both of these behaviours also increase the risk of binge eating. If you eat like this, you need to distribute your eating more evenly across the day using the regular eating procedure and healthy portion sizes. Your therapist can help you regularise your eating to maintain a stable and healthy energy intake.

Tackling the overvaluation of eating control

As we have mentioned, some young people with eating disorders overvalue eating control, not shape and weight control. These people often have an exceptionally high level of dietary restriction and restraint and tend to be particularly concerned about the precise details of eating. This is because they judge themselves mainly or even exclusively on their eating control. They repeatedly count calories and rigorously monitor nutrients they "should" be eating or avoiding (carbohydrates, fats and/or proteins). Some may even try to control their energy expenditure to this end.

If overvaluation of eating control is a problem that affects you, CBT-E recommends that you use the following procedures to address it:

- *Identify the overvaluation and think about its consequences*. This is approached using the same strategy for addressing the overvaluation of shape and weight in the Low Weight and Undereating module. You will draw up an extended formulation, which in this case will not include the typical expressions of the overvaluation of shape and weight (preoccupation with shape and weight, body checking, body avoidance or feeling fat), but rather those caused by the overvaluation of eating control. These are preoccupations with food and eating and food checking.
- *Enhance the importance of other self-evaluation domains*. This too involves the same strategies and procedures described in the Low Weight and Undereating module. You will be encouraged to develop other interests that take your mind and focus off eating control.
- *Reduce the importance of eating control*. The best way to do this is to address the expressions of your overvaluation. Specifically, food checking needs to be tackled using the strategies described earlier because it maintains preoccupation with food and eating. You should also avoid reading recipes and cookery books and stop looking at websites dedicated to food and eating.

Dealing with digestive complaints

Many people who fall into the trap of overvaluing eating control do so when they start to restrict their diet and avoid specific foods because they are experiencing digestive symptoms. They may feel bloating, nausea, abdominal pain, difficult digestion, constipation and/or diarrhoea, and limit what they eat in order to "cure" these symptoms. However, upon further investigation, in many people the onset of these symptoms can be traced back to a stressful situation. It is thought that the very act of restricting their diet is used to manage stress. Such people often feel the need to exercise self-control over various aspects of their life, like school, work, sports, other interests, and the restriction and avoidance of specific foods may give them relief from perceived failure in other areas of life.

Abdominal sensations generally go unnoticed, but if you are excessively focused on them, they may be experienced as digestive complaints. Although controlling your eating may relieve stress and lessen your fear of digestive complaints in the short term, when you start to lose weight, your digestive system won't work properly, and the digestive symptoms will proliferate and intensify.

If you have this problem, the strategy is to reduce your focus on these symptoms. Understand that they are the consequences of stress and low weight, not the amount or type of foods you eat. Remind yourself that once you start eating normally and restoring normal body weight these symptoms will go away. If you feel full, you should use the strategies described in the Low Weight and Undereating module to deal with this feeling. If you have difficulty managing the stress associated with your digestive symptoms, your therapist will be able to help you manage it without you restricting your diet or avoiding certain foods.

Of course, you may think that your digestive symptoms are down to a food intolerance. You may even have been told this by a practitioner of alternative medicine. However, you should know that in most cases the so-called food intolerance tests they use do not have a proven scientific basis, and what you are really suffering from is stress. To get to the bottom of this, your therapist should be able to put you in touch with a medical allergy specialist. Using validated scientific allergy tests, they will be able to tell you whether you are really intolerant to any food.

Fast Fact

Restriction and avoidance of foods without preoccupation with shape and weight are now considered symptoms of a new diagnosis: avoidant restrictive food intake disorder, more commonly known as ARFID. Whatever it is called, the transdiagnostic theory of eating disorders, and our clinical experience, tells us that CBT-E strategies and procedures can effectively treat it.

Alison's story

My life started falling apart about a year ago when I split up with my girlfriend. I guess I could have dealt with that, but I shattered my ankle the next day and had to give up my figure-skating career. So, I was 21, totally alone, miserable and no longer with any direction. Because I was basically immobile also, I started worrying about my weight. I developed lots of different rules about what, where and when I could and couldn't eat, and I'd hop down to the supermarket and spend hours looking at food packet labels. As soon as I had my cast off, I got really into rehab. I was determined to get back to peak condition and hoped I'd be able to make a comeback, even though the doctors had told me that with all the pins, my ankle would never be strong enough for me to compete. "Mind over matter," I thought, and threw myself into training. Unfortunately, this made me hungry all the time, and I ended up stuffing myself full of cake one night. I'd known I'd been losing weight, but I was okay with that—the lighter I got, the less weight my ankle would have to carry. I couldn't handle the idea that I'd just thrown away all my hard work and trashed my diet, though, so I booked an appointment with a psychotherapist. He helped me stop binge-eating, but I continued to lose weight, and I guess he got a little worried because he suggested I see a CBT-E specialist instead for a while.

That lady told me that it seemed to her that I placed too much importance on my body weight, and that healthy people aren't so afraid of putting on weight. She asked me whether I'd like to develop a more balanced view of things and stop having the starvation symptoms I'd been experiencing. What really gave me chills was when she explained to me that the likely result of depriving myself of important nutrients would be more fractures, so I agreed to give her way a go. I started regular eating like she suggested, but I guess I wasn't putting on as much weight as she expected, because she asked me about how I was eating. We ended up drawing up a really long list of my dietary rules, which went way beyond simple calorie counting. I weighed my food down to the precise gram, and then I'd weigh it again, just to be sure. I refused to eat certain food groups because I was petrified of putting on weight. I would never eat after 6 pm, and I would never eat anything that I hadn't made myself, because I wouldn't know what was in it. Of course, this made it impossible to have any kind of social life, and I kinda hoped to meet someone new one day, so I said that I'd do the Dietary Restraint module. I was also deathly afraid that my binge-eating episodes would start up again, and as my therapist explained, I realised that my extreme dieting would make them more likely.

That being said, I found it really tricky to introduce the foods I had been avoiding. We started off with one of the least threatening foods, full fat yogurt, but as soon as I ate any, my brain would be like: "Full fat?!? You broke a rule! You must eat less at the next meal." After discussing this with my therapist, we agreed that I was working myself up and risked jeopardising my own progress. The best thing for me to do was to work on my other dietary rules for a while, and try introducing avoided foods later on, when I felt ready to do so. In the end, I managed. I started off slow, with half a teaspoon of honey in my morning tea, and eventually I was able to rediscover my love of ice cream, without thinking too much about the calories it contains. Life is so much easier with a regular and flexible diet. It's great to be able to go out for meals with my friends again without the crippling anxiety.

In summary

The Dietary Rules module should help you tackle your extreme and rigid dietary rules. The strategies adopted by CBT-E for addressing dietary rules are as follows:

- Understanding that strict dieting is a problem—it damages your physical, mental and social health, and maintains your eating disorder.
- Identifying your dietary rules. You can do this by:
  - o Analysing the asterisks in your monitoring records
  - o Monitoring in real time to detect your dietary rules
  - o Considering if you have difficulty eating in certain situations and why
  - o Filling in the "Dietary Rules Inventory"
- Applying the strategy for addressing dietary rules in general:
  1. Identifying what is motivating a specific dietary rule
  2. Predicting the likely consequences of breaking the rule
  3. Breaking the rule on purpose
  4. Thinking about what happened when you broke the rule
  5. Planning further episodes of breaking the same rule until it is no longer a problem
- Addressing rules concerning when to eat (or rather when not to eat):
  1. Go to a supermarket and list all the foods you would be reluctant to eat.
  2. Score each avoided food on a scale of 1 to 4 based on the difficulty you would have eating them, and put them in groups.

3. Gradually introduce the avoided foods into your diet, starting with those that are least problematic.

The Dietary Rules module also includes specific strategies to help you:

- Manage your reactions to dietary rule-breaking
- Tackle food checking
- Tackle small meals and intermittent fasting
- Address the overvaluation of eating control

• Take-home message

By experiencing that the feared consequences of breaking dietary rules do not actually occur—you did not put on weight and you did not binge—you will gradually come to experience dietary rules as a problem rather than a helpful way of controlling your eating and/or body weight.

21

Events, Moods and Eating module

The Events, Moods and Eating module is for you if your eating behaviour is influenced by things that happen to you and how they make you feel. This link usually becomes more apparent when your treatment is underway, when you have already begun to address the major maintenance mechanisms of your eating disorder. Your mood is likely to have improved during CBT-E thanks to regular eating, reduction in dietary restriction and normalisation of body weight. However, if you are deviating from regular eating or having difficulty tackling your undereating and dietary rules in particular because of your mood swings, your therapist will suggest that you introduce this module.

This is because changes in eating triggered by events and associated mood changes are helping maintain your eating disorder (see Chapter 3 for details). They tend to create an obstacle to change that needs to be overcome.

Understanding if events and emotions are a problem

In Step Two, with your therapist, you will assess whether events and emotions seem to be fuelling your eating disorder. Let's say you deviate from regular eating or planned meals and snacks when something happens to you and/or your mood changes. These prompt recurrent binge-eating episodes, skipping meals and/or snacks and/or repeated episodes of self-induced vomiting or excessive exercising. If this is the case for you, it is a problem that needs to be addressed directly and effectively. First, you will learn how to deal with problems that you can see coming, and then those that you can't.

Tackling predictable events and emotions influencing eating

CBT-E suggests you use a specific proactive problem-solving procedure to learn to deal with the events and emotions that might potentially influence your eating. This procedure involves seven steps:

1. *Identifying the problem as early as possible.* Every time an event leads, or has the potential to lead, to a change in your eating, you should try to identify the underlying problem.

DOI: 10.4324/9781003342489-23

2. *Accurately specifying the problem.* This step requires a detailed reconstruction of the triggering event and how it affects your feelings, thoughts and behaviour. Common triggers include pressure at school, an argument or having nothing to do all day.
3. *Considering a range of possible solutions.* You should try to brainstorm as many potential solutions to the problem as you can think of, no matter how nonsensical or impractical they may seem. Even implausible solutions should be included on the list, as this may lead to identifying a previously unconsidered solution.
4. *Thinking through the implications of each solution.* You should examine the pros and cons of each of the potential solutions you thought of. What is likely to happen next?
5. *Choosing the best solution(s).* This step should be easy if the previous steps have been completed carefully.
6. *Putting the best solution(s) into practice.* The most crucial step in the problem-solving process is acting, applying the chosen solution(s). You don't need to be too inflexible in sticking to what you have planned—if it isn't working, try another potential solution from your list.
7. *Assessing the outcome.* Was your problem-solving a success? Think about how you applied the problem-solving procedure. This is more important than whether the problem was successfully overcome. Focus on developing their problem-solving *skills*. Try to get better and better every time.

To learn the procedure, it's best to practice. Think of a recent event that led to a change in your mood that influenced your eating. Your therapist will help you work through the proactive problem-solving procedure during a session. Then you should try to think ahead and identify potential issues before they arise. Each time you have a meal or snack, look ahead to the remainder of the day and try to predict when a problem and a change of emotion might occur. In this way your problem-solving becomes "proactive".

When you identify a potential a problem, you should do as Amina did in Figure 21.1:

1. Write "Problem" in column 6 of your monitoring record.
2. Turn over the page and practice problem-solving there and then (in writing).
3. Act on the solution identified.

The following day, think back to how you did in your problem-solving attempt and write your thoughts on the back of your monitoring record.

Problem-solving

Step 1—Identify the problem: Help! At a loose end

Step 2—Specify the problem: Jamie called me this morning to tell me that he cannot get out because he has a headache and fever. I'm disappointed because this Sunday afternoon I'm feeling a bit down and I wanted to go out with him. I am afraid because I do not have plans for the afternoon. I do not know what to do, I'm afraid of losing control. Plus, my aunt has just brought home a cake she made. It smells so good in the kitchen that I'm afraid to go in there. I think it's a risk.

Step 3—Options:	Step 4: Pros and cons:
a) Phone Francesca to go out	+ would make me feel better
	- she might not be able to come
b) Chat with my friends	+ would help me to relax
	- I can't message all the afternoon
c) Surfing the urge to binge without going out	+ It's about time for me to handle the urge without binging
	- I am afraid of giving in to the impulse to binge
e) Going for a walk in the park	+ would make me feel better and distract me from the smell of cake
	- I would be thinking about burning calories
f) Thinking about my parents' reaction if they found out I had binged	+ nothing
	- when I feel bad, I don't care what my parents think

Step 5 – Decide what to do: Options a, b, c are the best

Step 6 – Do it OK, 3 things: Call Francesca, then urge surf and chat

Step 7 – Review:

The best thing was I dealt with the problem immediately. I phoned Francesca, but she was not free. However, we set a date for next week. Messaging with friends helped me to relax and lifted my mood. It was also very helpful to see that I was able to handle the urge of binge eating. Yay! In the past, on afternoons like this I would certainly have binged.

Figure 21.1 Example problem-solving by Amina, who is using the strategy to overcome her urge to binge eat when she feels upset or gets bored

Handling unexpected events and emotions influencing eating

The systematic use of the proactive problem-solving procedure helps you prevent and cope with predictable mood changes due to events. However, emotions can also be triggered by unpredictable events. For this reason, you must use crisis management strategies to help you deal with the mood changes without changing your eating behaviour.

A helpful strategy in such cases is to apply the "things to say and do" procedure you learned about in Chapter 12. If this procedure is insufficient to get you over the hump, your therapist may suggest you address this problem with the Mood Intolerance module of the broad CBT-E form. The same module will be useful if you use some dysfunctional mood modulation behaviours like self-harming, drinking alcohol or other substances, to reduce your awareness of intense mood states and neutralise them.

Tackling residual binges

Binge eating is common among people with eating disorders, and it generally responds well and rapidly to the regular eating procedure implemented as part of Step One. If, however, you are still binge-eating in Step Two, try the procedures described in the following sections.

Preventing binge-eating wrecking your treatment

Most people with an eating disorder see binge-eating as a sign of their low willpower. They do not analyse and address the underlying maintenance mechanisms. This can lead to what we call the "control violation effect." This may occur when your behaviour (binge-eating) clashes with your goal (not having binge-eating episodes). This creates a conflict in your mind and feelings of guilt for having lost control, which could cause you to relapse and give up on treatment altogether. This kind of reaction is more likely if you blame your loss of control on a lack of willpower or personal worth, rather than a lack of skills. It is like throwing in the towel as soon as you first start learning to ride a bike. Say you fall off. Do you think it is because you will never be able to ride a bike, or because you haven't yet learned how to do so? To get any better, you need to get back in the saddle. Say to yourself that your binge-eating episode is only one step backwards on the road to recovery—a lapse, not a relapse. Relapse is defined by several repeated binge-eating episodes, not by one. One binge-eating episode is no big deal in the scheme of things. It is what you do now that will determine whether you recover or not. Get up, brush yourself off and start pedalling again.

Otherwise, the negative emotions caused by the conflict in your mind can lead to thoughts and behaviours that silence it. For example, after a binge-eating episode, a boy might think: "I will never get well. I am destined to be bulimic all my life. I may as well eat whatever I want and abandon any attempt to control my food intake." In this way, he no longer feels guilty after a binge-eating episode. If this was your friend, what would you tell them to do? Probably something like this, which is also what your therapist would suggest:

- Don't catastrophise if you have a binge-eating episode. It's not the end of the world—it's just a lapse, not a relapse.

- Don't blame low willpower for your binge-eating episode—it's just a lack of practice.
- Get back on track IMMEDIATELY. Do not fall into the trap of "taking a break" ("Since I failed to stick to my eating plan, I might as take the rest of the day off and eat what I want.") or compensating ("Since I ate too much at lunch, I'll skip dinner."). These two reactions make another episode of binge eating all the more likely.
- Do a *binge-eating analysis* (see next).

Binge-eating analysis

Say you have been free from bingeing for several weeks, and then one occurs. Binge-eating analysis has been designed to help you identify why. Immediately after any episode of binge-eating, ask yourself the following three questions:

1. Was the binge triggered by breaking a dietary rule?
2. Might I have been undereating over the last 24 hours?
3. Was the binge triggered by something that happened or how I felt?

You should do this every time it happens. The same strategy can be used to analyse any other deviations from regular eating you experience. It can be helpful to apply when you realise that you have been undereating for a while, skipped a meal or snack or experienced an episode of non-compensatory vomiting or exercising. Remember that if events and moods derail you, you should use proactive problem-solving to address triggering events.

Mindy's story

It sounds stupid now, but I started losing weight over a man. I was 22 years old, had a degree in economics, a good job and my own apartment, and what I thought was my forever guy. He, however, had other ideas about that, and told me he wanted to break up. He told me he hadn't but I convinced myself he had found someone new—someone thinner and prettier. I guess I had always been on the roly-poly side, but it hadn't really bothered me until then. After all, I had everything I wanted in life, and it wasn't as if I was a person with obesity! Restricting my diet gave me something to focus on, though, and I felt a great sense of achievement when I managed to lose the weight I wanted to. I felt powerful, no longer hopeless and unloved. However, I took it far too far and ended up being hospitalised because of my low weight. I spent a few months in an eating disorders unit and managed to put on a few pounds. They didn't get to the root of the problem though, because, as I realise now, the buzz I had been getting from losing weight I was now getting from gaining weight, so I effectively went too far in the other direction. I started stuffing myself between meals and ended up even heavier than I had been when this all started.

When I started CBT-E, I weighed 86 kg. I was extremely concerned about my shape and weight, and flip-flopping between bingeing and extreme dieting. I realise now that I was doing both to make myself feel better, but only ended up making myself feel worse. In all this, I'd managed to get me a new boyfriend, but he was no help: whenever he'd upset me or make a comment about what I was eating, I'd have a binge-eating episode and cry myself to sleep. Not the healthiest of relationships at the start, but that was mainly down to my eating disorder. In fact, the same thing would happen when I got a talking to from my boss. I was distracted all the time by thoughts of food, so I started making silly mistakes at work. When my boss pointed them out, I'd manage to keep it together until the end of the day, and then dissolve into a blubbery, chocolatey mess.

Although I'd done well up to that point, I was still having the odd binge-eating episode in CBT-E Step Two, so my therapist suggested we start the Events, Moods and Eating module, because every time I had a binge, it was a reaction to some emotional trigger. We worked on proactive problem-solving, and I learned to prepare for "at-risk" situations and how to handle them without binge-eating. My eating control is now much better, and I haven't had a binge-eating episode in months. I can now deal with my emotions much more effectively, and my relationship with my boyfriend is going from strength to strength!

In summary

The Events, Moods and Eating module is useful if events and associated mood changes influence your eating behaviour. If you find yourself binge eating, eating less or fasting after a troubling event, use the following strategies:

- Proactive problem-solving to handle predictable events and emotions influencing eating
- Things to say and to do to address sudden events and emotions influencing eating

If you have very intense emotions or dysfunctional mood modulation behaviours like self-harming, alcohol misuse or drug-taking, your therapist will teach you some procedures from the broad CBT-E Mood Intolerance module to manage them.

If you experience a residual binge, remember that it is a lapse, not a relapse. To prevent it derailing you your treatment, apply the following two strategies:

- Getting back in the saddle
- Doing a binge-eating analysis

• Take-home message

Events and moods can hijack your progress, but with practice and the right tools, you can learn to manage them effectively.

22

Setbacks and Mindsets module

Guided by your personal formulation, the strategies and procedures of Steps One and Two usually produce a marked reduction and often remission in the main eating-disorder features and expressions. You may no longer be troubled by low weight, dietary restriction and restraint, binge-eating episodes or excessive exercising, body checking and avoidance or feeling fat. As a result of the work you have done, the mechanisms responsible for keeping your eating-disorder mindset locked in place will gradually erode, progressively leaving time for healthier mindsets, appropriate for the circumstances, to be installed.

You may suddenly realise that you experienced no concern about eating or your appearance on a particular day, for example. This is evidence that your eating-disorder mindset is being displaced. At first these periods will be brief, because several different triggers may often activate the eating-disorder mindset. Once this happens, your eating-disorder features may rapidly return. The strategies of the Setbacks and Mindsets module will help you prepare for and prevent this happening.

Information on setbacks and mindsets

To understand what we mean by "mindset," it is helpful for you to think of your mind as a playlist. It contains different songs or videos labelled "friend," "son/daughter," "student," "athlete," "artist" and "musician," etc. Each song or video corresponds to a characteristic mindset that you switch on on specific occasions. For instance, at school, the "student" song will be playing. While spending the afternoon with friends, the "friend" song will start, and while in your parents' company, your "son/daughter" song is on. Under normal circumstances, you do this automatically. However, you also have an eating disorder, and therefore an "eating disorder" song. The problem is that this song does something strange to your software, and once you press play it gets stuck in a loop—you can't play any other songs, no matter what situation you are in. When you are at school, the "eating disorder" song comes on instead of the "student" song. When you are at sports practice, you can only play the "eating

DOI: 10.4324/9781003342489-24

disorder" song, and so on. In the same way, once you have an eating-disorder mindset, it tends to get locked in place, preventing you from seeing things as you normally would. By generating continuous concerns about weight, body shape and eating control, it makes it impossible for to concentrate fully on anything else. Your "eating disorder song" is all you will be able to hear, like an earworm—a song permanently stuck in your head.

In the later stages of treatment, once the main maintenance mechanisms of your eating disorder have been eroded, you will likely start to notice that there are times when the "eating disorder" song is not playing. The right song for the circumstances will start playing again. As a result, you may experience alternating states of being "in" or "out" of your eating disorder. At first, the "out" periods will be brief, because early on it is easy for the eating-disorder mindset to be reactivated. Once that happens, your eating-disorder features rapidly return (binge eating, dieting, vomiting, laxative misuse, exercising and/or body checking). Although thanks to this treatment, you have lessened the chances of the "eating disorder song" getting stuck in a loop, your eating-disorder mindset is very likely to reactivate in the initial stages of your recovery. This is the time to learn how to control your "eating disorder song," your eating-disorder mindset.

Controlling your eating-disorder mindset

The CBT-E strategy for controlling your eating-disorder mindset is the following:

1. Identify stimuli likely to reactivate your eating-disorder mindset (THAT song on your playlist)
2. Recognise the first signs that your eating-disorder mindset is reasserting itself (i.e., recognise the first bars of your "eating disorder" song)
3. Displace the mindset (by changing the track)

It is not a good idea to attempt this strategy in the early phases of the treatment because at that point, your eating-disorder mindset is firmly locked in place, and you have no other state to contrast it with. Once you start experiencing periods free from your symptoms and concerns, it will be easier for you to recognise and react when your "eating disorder" song comes on.

Identifying eating-disorder mindset reactivation triggers

In our experience, the most common events likely to trigger the eating-disorder mindset are the following:

- *Adverse shape or weight-related events*, like weight changes, clothes feeling tighter, mirror checking, feeling fat and receiving critical comments from others

- *Adverse eating-related events*, like eating an avoided food, eating "too much," binge-eating, feeling full
- *Adverse events in general*, like a bad school mark, a poor performance in a sports competition, being rejected or told off, etc.
- *Low mood*, brought on by unpleasant circumstances or an episode of clinical depression.

In order to spot the events and feelings most likely to trigger your "eating disorder song," you should monitor them real time. In most cases, such in-the-moment awareness is all you need to overcome the influence of these stimuli.

Spotting setbacks early on

There will inevitably be circumstances when your "eating disorder song" will reactivate. Sometimes, the first warning you get is changes in your eating behaviour. You might start restricting your diet or exercising excessively, or suddenly catch yourself body checking. These early warning signs are known as your "relapse signature"—the signal that you are sliding back down into your eating-disorder mindset. It is therefore essential that you immediately acknowledge that this is happening and take action to prevent it. Remember that when your eating-disorder mindset gets locked in place, you will find it all but impossible to change the tune. In fact, this can happen within a day or two, so you need to take action now. The quicker you react, the easier it will be to displace the eating-disorder mindset.

Displacing the mindset

In principle, there are two things you need to do:

1. "Do the right thing"—the thing you know you should do, not the thing your eating-disorder mindset is telling you to do
2. Engage in distracting activities with other people

"Doing the right thing" is easy, considering all you have learned in treatment about overcoming your eating disorder. Generally speaking, you should do the exact opposite of what the eating-disorder mindset wants you to. Instead of skipping a meal, eat a regular meal. If you get the urge to go for a second bike ride, have a nice, relaxing bath instead. It is helpful for you to do something fun or interesting to override these urges. Activities that involve other people, like going out with a friend, are usually the best, because having your "friend" track on will make it doubly difficult for your "eating disorder" song to start playing.

Practice makes perfect, and if you keep trying you will become increasingly adept at displacing your mindset. Successfully doing so will also make you feel good, as it creates a sense of mastery over setbacks. Although, as a rule, vulnerability to setbacks progressively declines over time, you need to retain this skill—you might need to use it in the future.

Exploring the origins of your overvaluation

Towards the end of treatment, it is helpful to explore with your therapist what may have triggered your sensitivity to shape, weight and eating. This exercise can help make you sense of how your eating disorder developed and evolved. In addition, it can highlight how your behaviour might have served a useful function in its early stages, and why it no longer does so. To help you review your past experiences (called a "historical review" in CBT-E terminology), your therapist will ask you to think about four distinct periods in your life:

1. Before the eating disorder (up to six months before its onset)
2. The six months immediately before its onset
3. The first months after its onset
4. The time since then

For each period, you should consider whether any events or circumstances might have sensitised you to your shape, weight or eating, or reinforced your existing concerns. You should then write down these events and circumstances in a *life chart*. Have a look at the example done by Ella in Figure 22.1. Using your life chart, talk to your therapist about why you think the eating disorder developed and evolved in the way it did.

Time period	***Events and situations***
Before the onset of the eating problem (until I was 14)	Mom and dad dieting Negative comments and criticism about my body shape from some schoolmates
The 6 months immediately before it started	COVID-19 lockdown and online lessons No ballet classes Loneliness and sadness My friend started a diet and using fitness apps
	Decided to go on a diet too
The 6 months after it started	Stuck to my diet and exercise plans perfectly Sense of total control Positive comments from my parents Rapid weight loss
From then till CBT -E	Cold intolerance, sleep disturbance, irritability, social isolation, poor concentration, and mood swings (at 15) Family therapy and antidepressants for one month (at 15½), but further weight loss Hospitalisation in a kids' hospital for low weight. Tube feeding to make sure I put on weight (at 15½).

Figure 22.1 An example life chart by Ella—although making a life chart cannot identify the causes of your eating disorder, it may help to talk about influential events with your therapist

Typically, events in the first period are of a type that might increase your awareness of your shape, weight and eating, perhaps a beauty pageant or a sporting competition, or like Ella, someone close going on a diet. You will probably find that in the second period (the six months leading up the onset) there will have been at least one stressful event or upheaval. In Ella's case it was the COVID-19 pandemic, but in yours it could have been moving from one city to another, changing school or jobs, your parents separating or the death of a relative. In the third period, when you started dieting, you probably had a feeling of being in control, which was a big relief after the destabilising event(s) that you experienced before. The fourth period is probably when the eating disorder became self-perpetuating—you were in the cycle, and the processes outlined in your formulation begin to operate. At this point, the eating disorder became more or less locked in place.

We cannot say for certain that the factors and processes you identified in your historical review operated in the way that you think they did. The object of the exercise is not to get a full explanation of your eating disorder—as we have said from the beginning, there are several factors involved, and we don't know exactly what they are. Nevertheless, reviewing the past in this way may help you distance yourself further from the problem and tends to enhance your understanding of the processes you are currently undergoing. We find that a historical review is particularly helpful in the later stages of treatment, when you can see that you are beginning to overcome your eating disorder. You may find, therefore, that it has a valuable "healing" function.

Balancing acceptance and change

A key step to decentring, taking a step back, from your eating-disorder mindset is for you to accept that the extreme weight-control measures you have been using do not actually work. Behaviours like strict dieting and/or excessive exercising do not help you to achieve the goal of maintaining a healthy weight and a natural body shape and can, in fact, destroy your life. Remember that weight and body shape are strongly influenced by genetics: it is possible to modify them partially, but the price to pay is to live forever with the adoption of strict and extreme dietary rules, starvation symptoms and persistent concerns about shape, weight and eating control.

You should weigh up the negative consequences of changing your natural shape and weight against the positives of maintaining a healthy weight, eliminating dietary restriction and restraint and your other unhealthy weight-control behaviours.

The goal is self-acceptance. This does not mean you have to love your body, but it is important to reduce its influence on the way you see yourself. A little body dissatisfaction is a normal part of life in the media-centric Western culture, but you should not let it run your life. Ideally, you should happily accept what your body naturally looks like, rather than just being resigned to it. It is easier to gradually accept your natural body weight and shape by stopping judging your body. Try to live with it as it is, without criticising it, scrutinising it or looking at it with contempt.

Other strategies for promoting body acceptance

Tackling the social pressure to be thin

It does not take much exposure to the Western media to realise the pressure on women to be slim and beautiful, and for men to be tall and muscular. Normal people who do not conform to these ideals are considered less attractive by some people. Cultural norms for physical appearance are difficult, if not impossible, for most people to achieve. A man might be able to make himself more muscular, but he is never going to get any taller. Body shape and weight too are partly controlled by your genes.

In Western societies, women in particular are pressured to be thin, because those who are thin are seen as not only more beautiful, but also more intelligent, competent and in control. This process of "positive thinness stereotyping" explains why many women and some men risk developing a self-evaluation scheme predominantly or exclusively based on their shape and weight. Other cultures, though, have different standards. Being overweight is a sign of prosperity and health in some Arab, African and Polynesian countries. Even in Western societies, the "ideal body shape" changes over time. What was considered attractive in the 1960s was totally different from what was considered attractive in the 1970s, for example. The wheel is always turning. The fact that beauty standards vary from country to country and within the same culture should tell you that the current norms are not objective or set in stone.

In addition to the general pressures, some people in Western societies are also under specific pressure to be thin or muscular. Examples include growing up in a family that places great importance on appearance and tends to criticise you if you put on weight, working in environments where there is an intense pressure to be thin or muscular (e.g., a clothing store or gym) or doing sports that require thinness (e.g., artistic gymnastics, running, etc.).

There are no ways to eliminate the general social pressure to be thin, and it can even be difficult to change specific social pressures. The thing to do, therefore, is to be aware of the problem and understand that extreme thinness is an unrealistic and unhealthy goal for people who are not genetically slim. Instead of taking it out on yourself, why not dedicate your energies to raising awareness of the issue? You might write a protest letter to a local newspaper about their publishing unhealthy messages from the diet industry or photos of emaciated models. You could join or set up a social media group to make a statement about weight stigma and the media pressure to be thin. In any event, you must not turn your dissatisfaction inwards. Try to reduce the emphasis on the psychological and social importance you attach to thinness. Remember that social stereotypes may influence whether you swipe left or right, but they have little importance in the development of lasting and satisfying interpersonal relationships.

Wearing comfortable clothes

Body checking and avoidance and feeling fat can be triggered by wearing clothes that are too tight. So, if your clothes are too tight, buy new ones that fit. Turn it into a fun shopping trip with a friend who can be trusted not to make unhelpful comments. Remember that your new clothes should not constrict you, but neither should they hide your body. What to do with your old clothes? Throwing them out or giving them to charity is a good way to distance yourself from your "eating-disorder self."

Managing comments on appearance

It is common after normalising weight to receive comments about your appearance. While your eating-disorder mindset might translate comments such as "You're looking well" or "You look good!" as "You look fat," know that this is not going to be the case. The person who made the comment really means it, and is probably very happy for you that you no longer look emaciated and ill. Accepting positive comments about your appearance is an essential step toward accepting your body. The normal thing to do when you receive positive comments is to smile, thank them and say something nice back. You should try doing the same.

Practising healthy physical activity

Healthy exercise can help you to accept your body shape and improve your mood. The decision on what type of physical activity to do should be carefully discussed beforehand with your therapist. They will talk you through the difference between exercise driven by shape and weight concerns and healthy exercise. The best physical activities for you require skills, socialising and some body exposure, rather than endurance. Try swimming or playing volleyball, tennis or golf with friends.

Oliver's story

I never liked my body much, and when I was 15, I began to get really into sports. My dad was a sporty person when he was younger, too, so I asked him for his advice on how to improve my performance. He suggested I follow a high-protein diet, and that seemed like a good idea. However, I got a bit fixated on both my diet and my training, and I lost a whole load of weight over the course of a few months. I was training every day for at least two and a half hours, and got to an all-time low weight of 45 kg. My parents got me into treatment, but that was based on the disease model of eating disorders, and I didn't get any better. This was how I ended up on CBT-E, which has helped me go into remission.

When I started, as well as low weight I had a morbid fear of weight gain, overvaluation of shape and weight and starvation symptoms. My diet was ridiculously strict and I was exercising excessively. Towards the end of Step Two, I had regained weight and significantly reduced my concerns about my body shape and weight. While I had had to stop basketball because of my illness, thanks to my treatment I was able to start it up again, just for fun. However, the dynamics of my team changed when several new players joined at the start of the new season. Things got really competitive, and one of my new teammates—I guess the star of the team—was talking about consulting a sports nutritionist, who advised him to eat carbohydrates on training days but not on resting days. I spent quite a lot of time thinking about this over the next few days and decided to follow this advice myself.

At first, I felt better, and my sports performance began to improve. But at the in-session weigh-in, my CBT-E therapist told me I had lost 2 kg. He tried to make me reflect on the dangers of weight loss, but I didn't see it as a problem—I was no longer underweight and in any case I felt great. What I did not understand at the time was that I had already fallen back into the trap. Over the next few weeks, my concerns about weight grew and grew, and I began to realise what was going on. My therapist explained to me that people with eating disorders are vulnerable to their eating-disorder mindset switching back on if they start trying to rigidly control their eating. He reminded me that the best way to control weight is through flexible healthy eating, and we started to work on a plan to deal with my situation, and to get ready for any future setbacks. I have to stay alert so I notice when my eating-disorder mindset kicks back in, and be ready to put in practice all the strategies I have learned for dealing with this. I now feel much stronger, because I know exactly what to do if my eating-disorder mindset starts to get the upper hand.

In summary

The Setbacks and Mindsets module is introduced towards the end of Step Two, once the main maintenance mechanisms of your eating disorder have started to crumble. At this point, you will likely start to notice that there are times when you are "in" your eating-disorder mindset and times when you are "out." In order to ensure that you stay "out," you need to learn how to control your eating-disorder mindset. The best strategy is the following:

1. Identify triggers that are likely to reactivate your eating-disorder mindset
2. Recognise when your eating-disorder mindset is coming back
3. Displace the mindset by "doing the right thing" or distracting yourself

Other strategies that may help you to decentre from your eating-disorder mindset are the following:

- Exploring the origins of your overvaluation using a life chart
- Balancing acceptance and change
- Handling the social pressure to be thin
- Wearing comfortable clothes
- Managing comments on your appearance
- Practising healthy physical activity

• Take-home message

If you to learn how to manage your eating-disorder mindset and any setbacks, you will be more able to stop yourself falling back into its trap.

23

Ending well

The end of the treatment is as important as the beginning

CBT-E, unlike other psychological treatments, which often simply fizzle out, places great importance on the final phase of therapy. For this reason, Step Three has been designed to help you end the treatment well. It has four main goals:

1. Addressing your concerns about ending treatment
2. Phasing out certain treatment procedures
3. Ensuring that you keep progressing
4. Minimising your risk of relapse in the long term

Step Three usually takes place over 3–4 sessions. The structure of the sessions does not change, but the sessions become progressively more future-oriented and less focused on the present.

Tackling concerns about ending treatment

While it is true that the treatment will soon end, this does not mean that your progress in overcoming the eating disorder has ended. Usually, you will continue to improve once the sessions have been wound up, and your concerns about shape and weight will continue to wane.

Only after a break from treatment, when you have had time to practice all the things you have learned without input your therapist, will it be possible for you to gauge just how much progress you have made. To fully recover, you will need to continue working hard over the following months, maintaining the changes you have made and striving for further progress.

Say you are learning a foreign language. In the beginning, you must rely on a teacher, and do a lot of homework. Then, after a while, if you want to improve and don't want to forget what you have learned so far, you will have to put your language skills into practice. You can do this by talking to people who speak that language and, if possible, going abroad to interact with native

DOI: 10.4324/9781003342489-25

speakers. In the same way, you need to practise and hone the CBT-E skills you have learned in the real world. This is why the treatment needs to end.

This does not mean you will be abandoned. Post-treatment review sessions will be scheduled 4, 12 and 20 weeks after your last session. This will give you and your therapist an opportunity to take stock of the situation and discuss any problems you may have been having.

Phasing out certain treatment procedures

Three sessions before the end of the treatment, you should stop doing monitoring in real time. It is neither realistic nor appropriate for you to continue monitoring yourself indefinitely. It is better to stop doing this while you are still in treatment, rather than at the very end, so you and your therapist can discuss any effects this interruption may have.

At this stage in the treatment, you will have already learned the skills you need to be more aware of your behaviours, thoughts and emotions as they happen. Therefore, monitoring—which is indispensable in the first two Steps of the programme—is no longer necessary. However, that does not mean you should take your eye off the ball. You need to watch out for potential problems. Keep an eye on how you eat and all other aspects of the eating disorder you have addressed during treatment (dietary rules, body checking and body avoidance, etc.).

Another procedure that you will stop at this point is in-session weighting. You should start to weigh yourself at home in the same way that you had previously been doing collaboratively with your therapist. Decide on a set day, once a week, and continue to keep a record on your weight chart. Remember to interpret your weight over a four-week span and not to fixate on the number on the scales. In the first few weeks of Step Three, however, weighing should be done both in-session and at home to calibrate the two scales. After that, you should begin to weigh yourself only at home and review your weight graph with your therapist.

Ensuring that progress is maintained

At the end of the programme, you may have some residual features of the eating disorder. This is to be expected. However, if you have interrupted the key maintenance mechanisms of your eating disorder, you should not worry too much about this. You will probably achieve full remission within a few months. That being said, it is best to be prepared, and so your therapist will help you draw up a plan to ensure you keep progressing.

Assessing the progress you have made

You can get a good idea of your progress by reflecting with your therapist on what has changed and what has not. However, it is best to do this review using a more systematic approach. Fill out the EPCL questionnaire and compare your scores with those you had at the start. It is also helpful to compare your last monitoring record with the one you did in first week of the treatment, and to draw an updated self-evaluation pie chart.

Look how far you have come! Be proud of the progress you have made. Although your therapist has helped you, only you are responsible for these changes.

Identifying features that you still need to address

You and your therapist will decide together which eating-disorder features remain to be tackled in the interval before the next post-treatment review. To identify these features, review your personal formulation. This should show you which residual features of the maintenance mechanisms still need to be dealt with.

Drawing up a short-term maintenance plan

Once you have identified the things you still need to work on, you will draw up a personalised short-term maintenance plan with your therapist. The plan will have two components:

1. *Continuing to "do the right thing."* You will be encouraged to do your best to continue behaving in the ways you have learned during treatment. You should continue to eat at regular intervals, weigh yourself weekly and keep an eye on your body checking, etc. If you don't, you will not obtain the full benefits of treatment. Remember that your treatment may have ended, but your recovery has not.
2. *Working on a limited number of residual features (up to four).* Examples of features typically targeted during the pre-review period include the following:
   - *Dietary restraint.* You will be asked to continue to introduce avoided foods and working on social eating, for example.
   - *Concerns about shape and weight.* This will involve trying out new activities and persevering with the hobbies you have taken up, as well as tackling residual forms of body checking and/or further body exposure, and continuing to reinterpret feeling fat.
   - *Events, moods and eating.* You must continue to practice proactive problem-solving—remember that practice makes perfect.
   - *Setbacks.* You will continue to work on identifying problems early, and practising displacing your eating disorder mindset.

The template shown in Table 23.1 can be used by you and your therapist to guide your personalised short-term maintenance plan. At the end of treatment, you will have a written copy of your personalised plan. Keep it to hand and look at it regularly to remind you to stay on track.

Table 23.1 Short-term maintenance plan template you can use to help you make a plan to address the residual features of the eating disorders

Eating disorder features	*How to address*
Dieting	• Avoid undereating. • Eat three meals and two snacks every day and not in between. • Eat a flexible and healthy diet. • Do not avoid social eating (i.e., with other people, in restaurants, etc.). • Do not avoid certain foods. • Avoid rigid and extreme dietary rules (e.g., a fixed number of calories, when to eat, eating less than others, to compensate for food already eaten or for a later meal). • Label feeling full as a normal and temporary sensation. If it becomes a problem, identify triggers (e.g., not being used to eating an average amount, being underweight, not eating regularly, wearing too tight clothing, eating an avoided food) and address them.
Other extreme weight-control behaviours	• Avoid vomiting/taking laxatives/excessive exercising • Other: . . . .
Concerns about shape and weight	• Weigh yourself only once a week and do not interpret single readings. • Stop problematic body checking (inappropriate clothing checks, pinching/touching, comparing self with others). • Use mirrors carefully. • Do not avoid seeing your body shape. • Be more aware of your body (e.g., by wearing different clothes; having a massage; etc.). • Identify the triggers of feeling fat and re-label. • Develop other life interests (e.g., ...). • Avoid judging yourself mainly on the basis of your shape and weight.
Binge eating	• Do a binge analysis to identify triggers (e.g., dieting, breaking a dietary rule, being underweight, going for too long without eating, alcohol, relaxing dietary control, events and emotions) and address them. • Use proactive problem-solving for predictable and recurrent high-risk situations. • Use the procedure of "thing to say and to do" to address sudden high-risk situations.
Weight maintenance	• Maintain weight within goal weight range (from . . . . to . . . .). • If the weight falls below this weight range → alarm bells! Review the pros and cons of weight regain, taking a long-term perspective. Remember you need to eat 500 extra calories daily to regain on average 0.5 kilograms a week. • Avoid any attempt to lose weight.
Other	• ____ • ____

Minimising the risk of relapse in the long term

Relapse is not uncommon following treatment for an eating disorder, and the period of greatest risk is the weeks and months following the end of treatment. To nip potential relapses in the bud, you must manage setbacks quickly and effectively. For these reasons, a fundamental goal of Step Three is to learning to minimise the risk of relapse in the long term. This builds upon and extends what you learned about dealing with setbacks in the Mindset and Setbacks module in Step Two.

General information on reducing the risk of relapse

Always keep in mind the following three points:

1. *It is important to have realistic expectations.* You should view your eating disorder as something that is still lurking around and may pop up and bite you at any time. No matter how far you have come, your eating-disorder mindset may slide back into your mind when you least expect it. However, as you will have learned in Step Two, this is something that you can manage.
2. *Some situations are riskier than others.* Situations that put you at risk of relapse include:

   - *Dieting.* If you restart strict dieting, break a major remaining dietary rule or have an episode of binge eating, you are more at risk of relapse unless you get straight back in the saddle.
   - *A change in your shape and weight.* If you put on weight, try on clothes that you think make you look fat, receive critical comments from others or experience shape and weight change following pregnancy, or weight loss due to illness, you need to be on your guard.
   - *Stressful circumstances or events.* Adverse events, especially those that threaten your self-esteem, can make you more vulnerable to falling back into your old ways.
   - *Clinical depression.* This may prompt you to stop eating or use dysfunctional mood modulation behaviours to make yourself feel better.

3. *It is crucial not to see lapses as relapses.* How you react to any setbacks will determine what happens next. You should view setbacks as mere lapses rather than a full-scale relapse, as this kind of black-and-white thinking will likely result in a self-fulfilling prophecy. Instead of passively resigning yourself to the hopelessness of it all, adopt a "can do" attitude to the problem, dealing with it as you have learned.

Strategy for dealing with setbacks

You need to develop a personalised plan for dealing with any setbacks. Essentially this should have two components:

1. *Spotting the setbacks straight away.* Avoiding wishful thinking and leap into action. "Do the right thing" and do something with friends to displace your eating disorder mindset as soon as possible.

2. *Analysing the trigger*. Take time out to think about what might have been the cause of your setback, and then address it using the problem-solving procedure you learned during treatment.

Your long-term maintenance plan

It is essential that you are well prepared to face the future. To this end, the last thing to accomplish is for you and your therapist to develop a written long-term maintenance plan. This will contain personalised advice on minimising the risk of relapse, including reminders on how to deal with triggers and setbacks. Table 23.2 can be used as a template for this purpose. You can adapt it to your specific needs.

Table 23.2 Long-term maintenance plan template you can use to make one of your own, to suit your specific needs

Minimise the risk of a setback

- Avoid dieting and the adoption of extreme and rigid dietary rules
- Eat three meals and two snacks every day and not in between
- Maintain weight within my goal weight range
- Don't do unhelpful body checking or body avoidance
- Maintain and develop other life interests
- Use problem-solving to tackle life problems

Events that might increase the risk of a setback

- Changes in daily routine
- Life changes and difficulties
- Weight loss or weight gain
- Depression or other psychological issues

Pay attention to the early warning signs of a setback

If you notice these early warning signs, react quickly by planning a course of action

- Eating less, skipping meals or snacks, eating "diet" foods
- Restarting diet
- Going back to looking at media focused on dieting and control of body weight and shape
- Restarting or increasing body checking or avoidance
- Weighing outside the once-a-week routine
- Increasing exercising
- Having the urge to vomit or use laxatives
- Having the urge to binge eat
- Increased concerns about food and eating
- Increased dissatisfaction with shape and weight, and a strong desire to lose weight
- Weight dropping below . . . . kg.

(*Continued*)

Table 23.2 (Continued)

Deal with triggers and setbacks

- Identify trigger
- Use proactive problem-solving
- Do not label a setback as a "relapse"—"get back in the saddle" straight away
- Restart using the key treatment procedures (real-time monitoring, weekly weighing, planning and adopting a pattern of regular eating, avoiding rigid and extreme dietary rules, binge analysis, "things to say and to do" and problem-solving for tackling problematic body checking or avoidance and feeling fat)
- Do the opposite of what the eating disorder mindset tells you to do—"do the right thing"; put effort into other aspects of your life, such as socialising—you decide the track you want to listen to
- Other:

- Other:

If the above has not worked within four weeks, consider seeking help.
If your body weight drops below . . . . kg for two consecutive weeks, seek help.

Post-treatment review sessions

Review sessions are usually planned 4, 12 and 20 weeks after the end of the treatment. These time intervals are short enough to give you something to work towards. At the same time, they are long enough to ensure that you have enough time to put your maintenance plan into practice and deal with the setbacks that will almost inevitably arise. The time intervals are also long enough so that you do not get confused about whether or not the treatment has ended.

The main purposes of your post-treatment reviews are the following:

- *To provide you with an opportunity to check in and report your progress.* It gives you a target to work towards.
- *To reassess your eating disorder.* This should be done in the usual way using the EPCL and other questionnaires.
- *To review how you are implementing your short-term maintenance plan.* You should review each point on your short-term plan with your therapist and whether they are still relevant.
- *To review how you have handled setbacks.* This is important. The goal is to perfect your problem-solving skills.
- *To decide whether there is a need for additional treatment.* You should talk to your therapist about whether your progress is being significantly affected by your residual eating-disorder features. If this is the case, a few

additional sessions should be enough to get you back on track after a setback and help you prepare to face any future setbacks.

- *To discuss the need for ongoing weekly weighing.* Whether you need to continue weekly weighing will depend on your attitude to your weight. If it remains an influential issue, you will be encouraged to continue the procedure, but if not, you can weigh yourself once every month or so.
- *To create or review the long-term maintenance plan.* Some new early warning signs of relapse or triggers may have emerged, and it is important that your long-term maintenance plan is updated with these in mind.

In most cases, the review appointments are positive occasions, and the 20-week post-review session will be the last time you need to meet with your therapist.

Alice's story

I remember being worried about my body shape and weight when I was 12. Then, when I was 13, I decided to become a vegetarian. I thought it would help me to lose weight, and it did, but later, when school started to get a bit stressful, the binge-eating began. As a result, my weight went up. During the first year of high school, a friend of mine went to see a nutritionist, so I did too. I started to follow some dietary rules and did more sports to help me lose weight, but I didn't have much success. I cut down even more on what I was eating and did more exercise. This helped me lose a bit of weight, but then the binge eating started up again, which I attempted to balance out by making myself sick afterwards. I was eating so little overall that my weight continued to drop, and when I reached 47 kg, my nutritionist advised an inpatient treatment. Being in hospital frightened me so much that I made a real effort to regain weight. I started eating more at meals, but this made me feel really out of control. So, when I was 17 years old and had a body weight of 58 kg I went for CBT-E.

At the start, I was fixated on my shape and weight. I was doing a really strict diet, as well as a ridiculous amount of exercising, bingeing and throwing up at least twice a week. CBT-E helped me get control of these behaviours, and my body weight gradually went up to 62.5 kg. At the beginning, I struggled to work on the mechanisms maintaining my eating disorder because I couldn't see losing weight as a problem. By then my whole life was about trying to change my body shape, and it was difficult for me to change my focus. However, I recognised that my binge eating was a problem, and so I agreed to tackle that. Getting over that hurdle made me feel more empowered, and I was ready for a new challenge. I agreed to stop trying to lose weight for a bit while I worked on my body image, and by the end of Step Two, I was far less concerned about my shape and weight and hadn't been bingeing and purging for weeks. I felt more in control of my eating, which was why I wanted treatment in the first place.

When I started Step Three, my therapist and I started looking to the future. At first, I was worried about weighing myself at home. I kept having flashbacks to before I started CBT-E, when I would weigh myself several times a day. I was I afraid I wouldn't be able to handle the urge to weigh myself more than once a week. However, I talked it through with my therapist, and she reminded me how important it was to have accurate information about my body weight and to understand that I was already an expert in interpreting my weight trend—not fixating on the number on the scales. This helped me to get over my fear and start weekly weigh-ins at home, just as we had done in the session. I continued to use my weight chart, and soon realised that weighing myself at home was easy. All I had to do was remind myself that it was pointless to weigh myself any more than that, because if I had put on or lost any weight, it would only be water weight, not actual weight. It's such a relief not to worry about my weight all the time.

In summary

CBT-E places great importance on the final phase of therapy. For this reason, Step Three has been designed to help you end the treatment well, and has four main goals:

1. Addressing your concerns about ending treatment
2. Phasing out certain treatment procedures
3. Ensuring that progress is maintained
4. Minimising the risk of relapse in the long term

Step Three usually takes place over 3–4 sessions, which become progressively more future-oriented and less focused on the present.

Three review sessions are planned 4, 12 and 20 weeks after the end of the treatment—these will give you something to work towards.

• Take-home message

Your recovery does not end when your treatment does. Nevertheless, the final phases of CBT-E will leave you in the best position to face the future with hope and confidence.

Part 3

Extra information

The broad CBT-E modules

Some people with eating disorders have more pronounced psychological and social problems that contribute to maintaining their disorder and interfere with treatment. We call these problems "non-specific" as people with other psychological disorders can also have them. The most common non-specific factors that can maintain eating disorders are the following:

- Clinical perfectionism
- Core low self-esteem
- Marked interpersonal difficulties
- Mood intolerance

The broad form of CBT-E has not yet been formally tested in young people with eating disorders. Therefore, we recommend using the broad form of CBT-E *only* when a non-specific eating-disorder maintenance mechanism meets all three of the following criteria:

1. It is pronounced.
2. It seems to be maintaining the eating disorder.
3. It appears to interfere with the response to treatment.

If more than one additional mechanism is identified, the one that seems to be contributing more to maintaining the eating disorder is chosen. Generally, though, the focused version should be used, because research into CBT-E in adults has found that the focused form is equally effective, but the broad is longer and more complex.

The decision to use the broad form of CBT-E is taken collaboratively with your therapist during the review sessions. Then, if you decide together that the broad form would be best for you, half of each session in Step Two will be focused on addressing the non-specific maintenance mechanism, and the other half the maintenance mechanisms specific to your eating disorder. For example, you might spend the first part of the session on your body image or dietary restriction, and the last half on your clinical perfectionism.

DOI: 10.4324/9781003342489-27

Detailed information on strategies and procedures used to address the additional maintenance factors can be found in the following books:

- **Clinical perfectionism:** Shafran, R., Egan, S., & Wade, T. (2018). *Overcoming perfectionism: A self-help guide using scientifically supported cognitive behavioural techniques* (2nd ed.). London: Little, Brown Book Group.
- **Low self-esteem:** Fennell, M. J. (2016). *Overcoming low self-esteem: A self-help guide using cognitive behavioural techniques* (2nd ed.). London: Little, Brown Book Group.
- **Marked interpersonal difficulties:** Albert, R., & Emmons, M. L. (2017). *Your perfect right: Assertiveness and equality in your life and relationships* (10th ed.). Oakland, CA: Impact Publisher.
- **Mood intolerance:** Van Dijk, S. (2021). *Mood intolerance: The DBT skills workbook for teen self-harm: Practical tools to help you manage emotions and overcome self-harming behaviours*. Oakland, CA: New Harbinger Publications.

25

Distance CBT-E

When face-to-face sessions are not possible, you can ask to receive CBT-E online. The COVID-19 pandemic prompted the governments of many countries to recommend social distancing. As a result, psychological treatments for patients suffering from eating disorders were difficult to access. This situation required a new way of providing psychological treatments for eating disorders, since psychotherapy in the therapist's office was not practicable.

The solution to this problem, at least in part, was to adapt CBT-E so it could be used on the various video-calling platforms. The promising results obtained with this new mode of delivering CBT-E have opened up new perspectives on the possibility of its practical use, even for people who have difficulty attending face-to-face sessions under normal circumstances, or for people living in places where specialised services for the treatment of eating disorders or the psychological treatments recommended by international guidelines are not available.

CBT-E is well suited for distance therapy

CBT-E is readily adapted for teletherapy. The patient and therapist can easily talk remotely via online video-calls. There is not yet any data on distance CBT-E, but developing an excellent collaborative therapeutic relationship and delivering most aspects of treatment is possible. In our experience, virtual sessions do not compromise most of the non-verbal communication aspects of the therapeutic relationship.

Effectiveness of distance therapy

Although research is still limited, the initial data on delivering other psychological treatments through video-calls suggests that assessments and therapy sessions can work well using this mode of delivery. Promising results for using distance therapy to treat depression and generalised anxiety have been reported. CBT for bulimia nervosa delivered via telemedicine is reported to be acceptable to patients, and roughly equivalent to face-to-face delivery.

DOI: 10.4324/9781003342489-28

Delivering distance CBT-E

Delivering CBT-E remotely is possible using various video-calling platforms (e.g., Zoom, Skype, Meets, etc.). The choice will depend on multiple factors, including the preferences of you and your therapist, your internet service providers, how well the platform functions with the available bandwidth and legal issues such as such as confidentiality. Video-calling platforms are best, because it is not possible to share materials live onscreen or observe non-verbal communication through audio calls.

In many cases, it is possible to send therapy documents like your self-monitoring records electronically. If it is impossible to share these materials securely, alternative solutions may be found. For example, you could tell your therapist what you wrote.

Challenges of distance CBT-E

If you choose to receive this mode of therapy, you will have to work with your therapist to consider and overcome any obstacles. For example, distance therapy may produce particular challenges if you are not already familiar with the technology and have little privacy at home.

If you can't stop checking your appearance on a video-calls, your therapist could help you consider the ways different platforms allow you to hide yourself and only view the therapist. However, video-calls can be an opportunity for you to build up a tolerance for viewing yourself and practising ways of not checking your appearance in an unhelpful manner. Building such a tolerance is important, as otherwise, this could create problems for you in other forms of virtual socialising.

Many of the challenges of this form of delivery can be relatively easily overcome if you work with a therapist with whom you have already developed a trusting relationship during initial face-to-face treatment. It might be more challenging if the treatment is delivered remotely without any initial face-to-face contact, since it might be more difficult to develop a collaborative relationship.

Advantages of distance CBT-E

Remote therapy has clear advantages, too. For you, it is often more convenient, less disruptive to daily life and may be less costly. It also occurs in the same place you spend your time, potentially avoiding a context-dependent change only. It may also mean that twice-weekly sessions, where appropriate, are easier to put into practice.

CBT-E emphasises the importance of you working on specific tasks between sessions to bring about change. This is perfectly consistent with working remotely. Indeed, with distance therapy, it is easier for you to see that it is you who is making the change, rather than your therapist.

Main adaptations of distance CBT-E

Sessions will usually be the same length as face-to-face sessions. However, there could be a break in the middle if a full session is not feasible. Distance CBT-E adopts the same strategies and procedures as face-to-face CBT-E, but with some adaptations. These are described below.

Learning what treatment will involve

As in face-to-face CBT-E, in the preparation sessions, your therapist will describe the treatment in detail and seek to actively involve you. Compared to conventional CBT-E, however, some additional topics must also be addressed. These include assessing your attitude towards this mode of therapy and the practical aspects of online sessions. You will need to decide together upon the video-call platform to be used, the possibility of being able to carry out the sessions without interruption in a closed room and how to deal with any loss of internet connection.

Jointly creating the personal formulation

In face-to-face CBT-E, the therapist draws the formulation diagram on paper. In the remote session, your formulation can be drawn using the digital whiteboard provided by the video-call platform or on paper that must be scanned/photographed and sent to you. Then you should print it and put it on your table so that you can always have an eye on it during distance sessions. Whether in-person or digital, the formulation will always be created collaboratively, with input from both the therapist and you.

Establishing real-time self-monitoring

During in-person sessions, the therapist explains and gives you copies of blank self-monitoring records. In remote CBT-E, your therapist should send you a blank copy of the monitoring record via the platform's chat function. Then, you should print it at home and fill in your monitoring records using pen and paper. If you do not have access to a printer, you can create monitoring records on paper by drawing the same columns used on the CBT-E monitoring record.

As with in-person CBT-E, your monitoring records are reviewed collaboratively with your therapist at the beginning of each online CBT-E session. For this reason, you must send them a photo or a copy of your monitoring records by email or via the video-call platform (bearing in mind security and confidentiality issues) before the start of each session.

Collaborative weighing and weight chart

Your therapist is responsible for preparing and keeping your weight chart, and then sharing it with you during the session. During in-person sessions, you and your therapist will conduct the weighing in session and review your weight chart together. This will not be possible in a distance setting, but there are a couple of remote options. Firstly, it may be possible for you to move your video-call device so that the therapist can be present and see the actual weighing process. This will allow the therapist to maintain the weighing procedure as close to standard in-person treatment as possible. Alternatively, you could weigh yourself before or during the session while the therapist waits for your report. It is vital that you give an honest report on the number on the scales.

Using this treatment guide

In CBT-E delivered in person, your therapist will provide you with or ask you to buy this book during the preparation sessions. In remote CBT-E, your therapist can indicate where you can buy this book on the internet or send it to you by mail (if they have copies available).

This guide's "guided reading" is used to educate you about eating disorders and how to use the CBT-E strategies and procedures optimally. It does not require any modification when delivered remotely.

Establishing regular eating

This procedure requires no modification from standard CBT-E to be implemented remotely, as all the practical application takes place between sessions. The goal is still that you eat at regular intervals throughout the day, having three meals and two snacks and not eating in between.

Deciding to tackle weight regain (if applicable)

This procedure does not require modification from standard CBT-E. After drawing up and discussing your personalised pros and cons of change tables, you and your therapist will collaboratively draw a conclusions table with your reasons/incentives to change. These tables will be created during the CBT-E session, either through the screen-sharing whiteboard option or on paper with the webcam.

Review sessions

Distance CBT-E uses the same review sessions, strategies and procedures as standard CBT-E. The identification of any existing barriers to change should also include assessment of your attitudes towards distance treatment and the use of online CBT-E procedures.

Tackling undereating and being low weight, dietary restraint, excessive exercising and purging

These procedures don't require any change from standard CBT-E. You will be actively involved in planning meals and snacks to create a positive energy balance of 500 kcal. This increased number of calories should enable an average weight regain of 0.5 kilograms per week. If you adopt strict dietary rules, CBT-E encourages flexibility. Addressing rigid and extreme dietary rules, excessive exercising and purging remotely do not require significant modification from standard CBT-E.

Tackling body image

This procedure doesn't require modification from standard CBT-E. Work on increasing the importance of other domains of life, addressing shape checking and avoidance and feeling fat, can be done via webcam.

The same strategies and procedures implemented in face-to-face sessions can be used to address shape avoidance and feeling fat. The monitoring records reporting shape checking can be easily filled in and reviewed during distance CBT-E, and comparison making homework activities, such as comparison monitoring, researching online examples of body image manipulation (airbrushing and similar) and sitting somewhere public, like a café (if allowed), actively looking at the body of every third person you encounter (or can see out of the window), can all be done from home.

Dealing with events and moods

Events and associated mood changes may negatively influence your eating and should be addressed using standard CBT-E procedures, which can be delivered remotely.

Handling setbacks and mindsets

Your eating disorder can be viewed as a "mindset." In CBT-E, you learn about mindsets and how to recognise, control and replace them. The same strategies and procedures used to achieve this during face-to-face work can be employed when delivering CBT-E remotely.

Broad CBT-E modules

The broad form of CBT-E is designed only for patients in whom mechanisms external to the eating disorder features also contribute to maintaining their eating disorder and preventing change. All the external maintenance mechanisms (i.e., clinical perfectionism, core low self-esteem, marked interpersonal difficulties and mood intolerance) can be addressed remotely using the same strategies and procedures as standard CBT-E.

Handling the end of the treatment

The last step of the treatment, as per standard CBT-E, should be focused on ending treatment well. It is possible to use the usual strategies and procedures when delivering this intervention remotely.

Post-treatment review sessions

Review sessions are planned 4, 12 and 20 weeks after the end of the treatment and do not require any modification from standard CBT-E.

Parental involvement during remote CBT-E

Your parents can be very helpful in supporting you with distance CBT-E. As with in-person CBT-E, the role of your parent will still be as a "helper," and how much or how little support they will be asked to provide will be decided in conjunction with you.

As in standard CBT-E, distance CBT-E includes one 50-minute session with parents alone and several 15- to 20-minute joint sessions that parents join at the end of a patient's individual session. Both of these types of sessions can be conducted online. Remote CBT-E uses the same strategies and procedures adopted by standard CBT-E to involve your parents in creating an optimal family environment and supporting you in implementing some treatment procedures.

Further reading

Dalle Grave, R. (2020). Distance CBT-E for eating disorders in light of COVID-19. *Psychology Today*. Retrieved from www.psychologytoday.com/intl/blog/eating-disorders-the-facts/202004/distance-cbt-e-eating-disorders-in-light-covid-19

Murphy, R., Calugi, S., Cooper, Z., & Dalle Grave, R. (2020). Challenges and opportunities for enhanced cognitive behaviour therapy (CBT-E) in light of COVID-19. *The Cognitive Behaviour Therapist*, *13*, e14. doi:10.1017/s1754470x20000161

26

Final thoughts

We hope that this book has given you a better understanding of your eating disorder and the procedures you will use to overcome it. The road will be a long and sometimes hard one, but there is real hope that through CBT-E you can become a happy, healthy young person and go on to have a fulfilling life.

Best of luck!

Riccardo and Simona

DOI: 10.4324/9781003342489-29

27

Resources

CBT-E website

www.cbte.co

The website provides up-to-date information on CBT-E and guidance for identifying suitable CBT-E-trained professionals around the world.

Academy for Eating Disorders

Founded in 1993, the AED is a global professional association committed to leadership in eating-disorder research, education, treatment and prevention. The goal of the AED is to provide global access to knowledge, research and best treatment practice for eating disorders. It also provides links to other similar organisations in the United States and abroad: www.aedweb.org.

Other useful links

www.nhs.uk/conditions/eating-disorders/
www.mind.org.uk/information-support/types-of-mental-health-problems/eating-problems/types-of-eating-disorders/
https://kidshealth.org/en/teens/eat-disorder.html www.nationaleatingdisorders.org

DOI: 10.4324/9781003342489-30

28

CBT-E tools

Table 28.1 My Monitoring Record

*Day*________________________ *Date* ________________________

Time	*Foods and drink consumed*	*Place*	*	*V/L/E*	*Context and comments*

Note: V = vomiting; L = laxative misuse; E = exercise.

Source: Reproduced with permission from Online Training Program in CBT-E, CREDO Oxford, 2017.

DOI: 10.4324/9781003342489-31

Table 28.2 My Monitoring Record For Shape Checking

*Day*____________________ Date____________________

Time	*Food and drinks consumed*	*Place*	*	*V/L/E*	*Check (type, time)*	*Context and comments*

V = vomiting; L = laxative misuse; E = exercise

Table 28.3

MY WEIGHT CHART

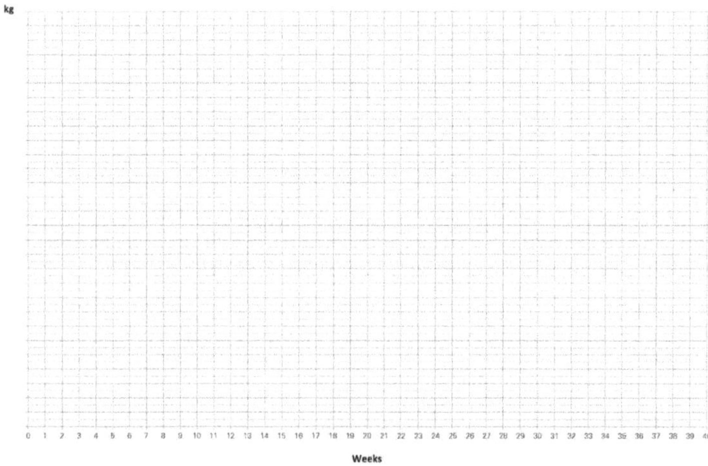

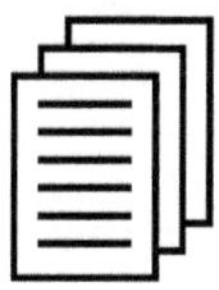

Table 28.4 Eating Problem Check List (Epcl) 3.1

INSTRUCTIONS: The following questions are concerned with the past seven days only. Please read each question carefully. Please answer all the questions. Thank you.

In the past seven days . . . *(indicate the number of times that this has occurred in the box on the right)*	*No. of episodes*
Have I eaten a large amount of food with a sense of having lost control (i.e., an objective binge-eating episode)?	
Have I eaten a not large amount of food with a sense of having lost control (i.e., a subjective binge-eating episode)?	
Have I made myself sick (vomited) as a means of controlling my shape and weight?	
Have I taken laxatives as a means of controlling my shape and weight?	
Have I taken diuretics (water pills) as a means of controlling my shape and weight?	
Have I exercised excessively as a means of controlling my weight, shape or amount of fat, or to burn extra calories?	
Have I weighed myself?	

In the past seven days . . . *(tick which box is true for you)*	**0 Never**	**1 Rarely**	**2 Sometimes**	**3 Often**	**4 Always**
Have I avoided some foods as a means of controlling my weight, shape and/or eating?					
Have I reduced my food portions as a means of controlling my weight, shape and/or eating?					
Have I checked my food (e.g., calorie counting, weighing food, checking the food's nutritional content)?					

Table 28.4 (Continued)

In the past seven days . . . *(tick which box is true for you)*	**0 Never**	**1 Rarely**	**2 Sometimes**	**3 Often**	**4 Always**
Have I checked my shape (e.g., looking at parts of my body in the mirror; measuring the circumference of parts of my body; compared my body shape with that of other people)?					
Have I avoided my body (e.g., avoided weighing, avoided particular clothes, avoided looking at my body)?					
Have I felt fat?					
Have I been preoccupied with my weight?					
Have I been preoccupied with my shape?					
Have I been preoccupied with my eating control?					

Table 28.5 Eating Problem Check List (Epcl) Summary Sheet

Date																				
Week																				
Body weight (kg)																				
Objective binge eating																				
Subjective binge eating[1]																				
Vomiting[1]																				
Laxatives[1]																				
Diuretics[1]																				
Excessive exercising[1]																				
Weight checking[1]																				
Food avoidance[2]																				
Reduction of food portions[2]																				
Food checking																				
Body shape checking[2]																				
Body avoidance[2]																				
Feeling fat[2]																				
Weight preoccupation[2]																				
Body shape proeccupation[2]																				
Eating prepccupation[2]																				

[1] Number of events at the last seven days

[2] 0 = never, 1 = rarely, 2 = sometimes, 3 = often, 4 = always

Table 28.6 Dietary Rules Inventory (Dri)

The following questions cover the last four weeks (28 days). Read each question carefully and put a tick in the appropriate box.

How many times over the last 28 days have you intentionally tried					
	Never	*Rarely*	*Sometimes*	*Often*	*Always*
1. Not to eat after a certain time					
2. To delay mealtimes					
3. To eat the same foods					
4. Not to eat outside of main meals					
5. To eat the lowest calorie foods					
6. To eat less than the others with you					
7. Not to eat in front of other people					
8. Not to eat when meeting up with other people					
9. Not to eat foods considered fattening					
10. Not to eat foods considered unhealthy					
11. Not to have dessert at the end of a meal					
12. Not to drink sugary drinks					
13. Not to use condiments					
14. Not to eat foods whose ingredients, calorie content or precise quantity are unknown					
15. To restrict previous meals if you plan to eat away from home					
16. Not to accept invitations to lunch or dinner					

(Continued)

Table 28.6 (Continued)

How many times over the last 28 days have you intentionally tried					
	Never	*Rarely*	*Sometimes*	*Often*	*Always*
17. Not to eat certain food groups (e.g., carbohydrates, fats, proteins, other)					
18. To cook separately from others					
19. Not to eat food prepared by others					
20. Not to eat condiments left on the plate					
21. To leave pieces of food on the plate					
22. Not to have seconds					
23. Not to eat if you haven't burned enough					
24. Not to taste food while cooking					
25. To establish a fixed calorie limit for the day					
26. To establish a fixed calorie limit for an individual meal					
27. To establish a fixed number of pieces of food to eat					
28. To have small portions					

Index

Note: page numbers in *italics* indicate a figure and page numbers in **bold** indicate a table on the corresponding page.